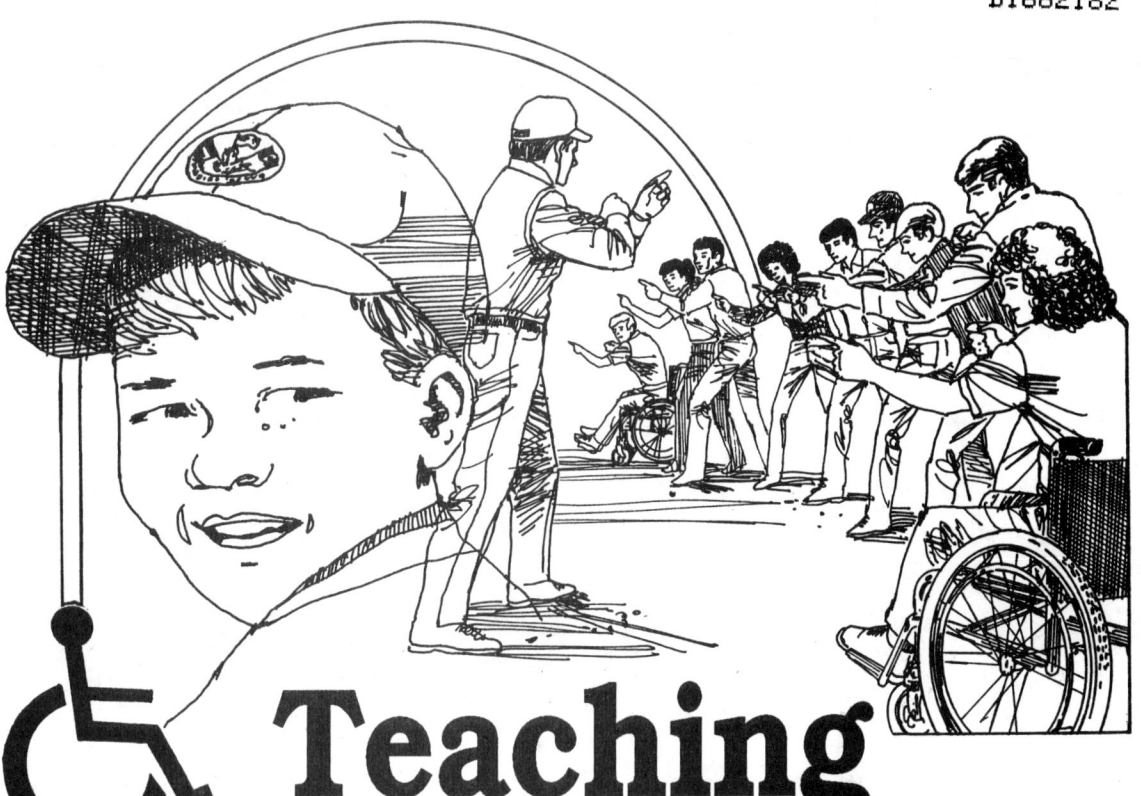

# Teaching Shooting Sports
## to persons with disabilities

Outdoor Empire Publishing, Inc.
Seattle, Washington

Copy Editors: Robin Taylor, Dennis Carpenter, and Dave Workman
Cover Design: Tex Wilson
Art: Tex Wilson
Type and Page Composition: Judy Richardson, and A. Taylor
Project Director: Maureen Liang

Library of Congress Catalog Card number: 93-49380
ISBN: 0-916682-66-8
Stock number: 1090-63

Printed in the United States of America

Copyright © 1994 by Outdoor Empire Publishing, Inc.
All rights reserved. No part of this book may be reproduced
in any form or by any process without permission in writing from the publisher.

Manufactured by Outdoor Empire Publishing, Inc.,
P.O. Box C-19000, 511 Eastlake Avenue East, Seattle, WA 98109.
Phone: (206) 624-3845
FAX (206) 340-9816

Lesson Plans on pages 27-36, 41-50 and 57-65 may be duplicated for use by the instructor
in the instructor's classroom. They may not be reproduced for sale or mass distribution.

Outdoor Empire Publishing, Inc. is not responsible for any adverse effects or consequences
from the misapplication or injudicious use of the information contained within this text.

*Equal opportunity to participate in and benefit from hunter education programs is available to all individuals without
regard to their race, color, national origin, sex, age, or handicap. Complaints of discrimination should be sent to the
Office of Equal Opportunity, U.S. Department of Interior, Office of the Secretary, Washington, D.C. 20240.*

# Acknowledgements

The publishers would like to thank the Missouri Department of Conservation, which produced the original text for this manual, and without whose continued assistance, the finished version would not have been possible.

Some portions of this publication were printed with permission by The Center for Recreation and Disability Studies in the Curriculum in Leisure Studies and Recreation Administration at the University of North Carolina at Chapel Hill; Publications: *LIFE RESOURCES, The LIFE Resource Manual,* and *LIFE FORMS, The LIFE Training Guide.*

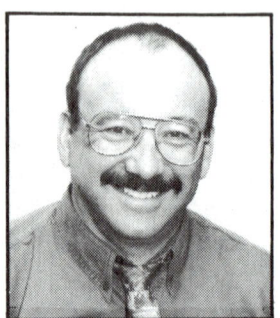

**JEFF PAGELS** of the Wisconsin Department of Natural Resources has been a District Community Services Specialist since 1974. He has extensive involvement in Disability programs, and he also does volunteer peer counseling at St. Vincent Hospital in Green Bay. He developed a park and recreation accessibility manual and served as chief advisor in the preparation of a video on accessibility. He is an accomplished disabled cross-country skier and athlete, having represented the U.S. in Norway twice and in South America in a 1990 swimming competition. He has received several awards, and he is one of the first two wheelchair athletes to successfully complete the dangerous Sierra-Nevada cross country ski crossing.

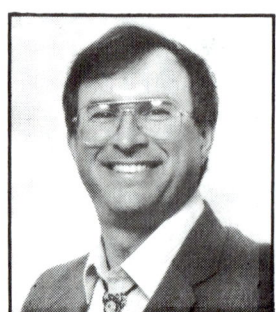

**RICK JULIAN** is a biologist with the U.S. Fish & Wildlife Service. His career has spanned more than 20 years, during which he has held positions as Regional Hunter Education Specialist and Regional 504 compliance officer. He is the Wildlife Team Leader for the Federal Aid Division in Fort Snelling, Minn. Julian organized and lead a team in the design and development of the video *Access for Everyone* for the FWS.

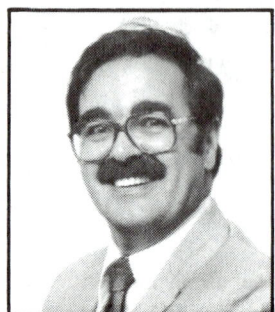

**JAMES A. DABB** served with the Michigan Department of Natural Resources' Law Enforcement Division until his retirement in 1991. He is a hunting safety and firearms safety expert witness, and still serves as a volunteer Hunter Education instructor. He was the one-time Hunter Education coordinator for Michigan, and recipient of the Hunter Education Association Hall of Fame Award. He developed materials and teaching aids for use in programs in his state, and across North America. He also served as a consultant on four films/videos and two student workbooks. He established an annual week-long Volunteer Instructor Academy for the Michigan Hunter Education instructors program, and he still serves as an instructor at this academy.

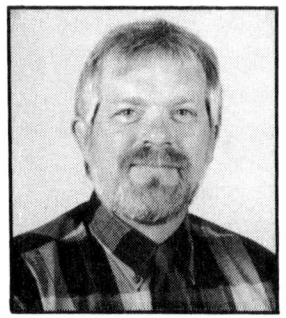
**RICHARD L. FLINT** taught secondary education for three years in the Missouri public school system before taking a position with the Missouri Department of Conservation as an Outdoor Skills Specialist. Rick has presented formal programs for the disabled before several groups of Hunter educators. He is presently assigned to the MDC's Southwest Protection region as a Hunter Skills Specialist and is actively involved in shooter education programs. He has also been involved in teaching classes for the Therapeutic Recreation Department at Southwest Missouri State University.

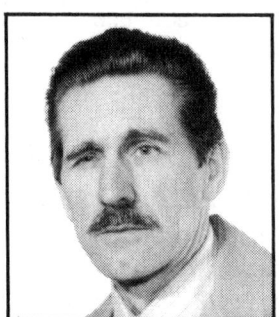
**GARY ANDERSON** has been a safety officer with the Maine Inland Fish & Wildlife agency, where he serves as the Hunter Education administrator. He is a recipient of the Hunter Education Association Hall of Fame Award, and an advisor to the Board of Directors of Disabled Outdoor Experiences (DOE) of Jackman, Maine. He is co-author of *Maine Outdoor Recreation for Everybody*. Gary also served as search and rescue coordinator for Maine from 1980 to 1991, and sits on the Board of Directors for the National Association for Search and Rescue.

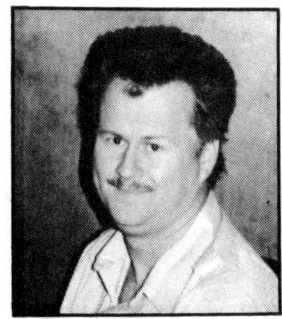
**RAY WELLER** of Stayton, Ore. was the Winchester Hunter Education Instructor of the Year for 1990. As volunteer state coordinator for Oregon's Hunter Education program, Weller has trained and evaluated more than 250 instructors. He was instrumental in establishing Hunter Education classes for the hearing impaired, and also bird hunting programs for wheelchair sportsmen. He is a founder of the Oregon Hunter Education Instructors' association and a member of the Beaver State's Shooting Sports Program Fund Committee. He has also served as an HEA associate board member.

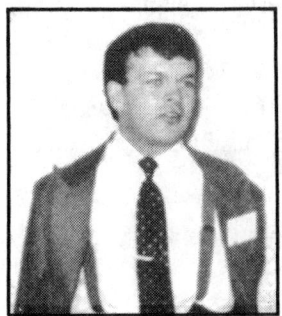
**MICHAEL NOYES** is a certified elementary school teacher in Maine, where he works part time for U.S. Senator William S. Cohen. He is also employed by the Pine Tree Society for Handicapped Children and Adults in the community of Bath. He grew up in rural Maine, the eighth of twelve children. Noyes coaches soccer and is a volunteer fund raiser for the Pine Tree Society's summer camp program. He also works with snowmobilers and other sports-oriented groups. Noyes holds a degree in rehabilitation and psychology from the University of Maine.

# Chapter Organization

**Guideline for Disabilities**

This section discusses various levels of ability, and what limitations each level places on an individual. There is advice on dealing with physical, mental, learning, hearing and visual impairments.

**Disability Awareness**

Students with different abilities require differing levels of assistance. This section offers an overview dealing with various abilities, and helps the instructor be aware of some needs related to specific impairments.

**Access for All People**

This section discusses various means of assisting students with disabilities in overcoming obstacles that may be taken for granted by those without disabilities. There are tips on wheelchair accessibility, and adapting both the program and the environment to accommodate all students.

**Instructor and Student Safety**

A detailed look at common sense steps to assure safe range conditions for students and instructors. Not only are there tips on making the program safe, but also on making the environment safe.

**Teaching Students with Disabilities**

This section addresses sport opportunities available across North America to people with disabilities. It also offers some advice on how to make the most of their time in the outdoors.

**Rifle/Airgun Theory & Assistive Devices**

There are many assistive devices to help shooters overcome their disabilities for various levels of shooting. This section covers airguns, small- and large-bore rifle and pistol shooting, and assorted assistive devices available. There is also a riflery lesson plan.

**Shotgun Theory & Assistive Devices**

Like the previous section, this segment deals with shooting. Specifically, this section addresses shotgun shooting, the options available for shooters and some of the assistive devices that can be employed. A shotgun lesson plan is included.

**Archery Theory & Assistive Devices**

Archery is one of the toughest hurdles for some disabled persons. This section addresses those problems with discussions of various types of bows and assistive devices. An archery lesson plan is included.

**Appendices**

These are designed to offer support information to the reader, and other resources to which the reader can refer. Included are state-by-state details on what the states are offering for disabled sportsmen and women.

# Table of Contents

## 1. Guidelines for Disabilities    3

    Physical Impairments    4
    Mental Impairments    4
    Learning Impairments    4
    Hearing Impairments    5
    Visual Impairments    5

## 2. Disability Awareness    7

    Students with Physical Impairments    7
    Students with Hearing Impairments    8
    Students with Visual Impairments    9
    Students with Mental Impairments    11
    Students with Learning Impairments    12

## 3. Access for All People    13

    Wheelchair Pointers    13
    Change of Environment    14
    Change the Program    14

## 4. Instructor and Student Safety　　15

Range Procedure Tips　　15
Program Safety　　17
Environmental Safety　　17

## 5. Teaching Students with Disabilities　　19

Some Tips　　19
Hunting Opportunities for
　People with Disabilities　　20

## 6. Rifle/Airgun Theory & Assistive Devices　　21

Airguns　　21
Small Bore & Large Bore Rifle and Pistol　　22
Assistive Devices　　22
Riflery Lesson Plans　　27

## 7. Shotgun Theory & Assistive Devices    37

| | |
|---|---|
| Shotguns | 37 |
| Other Shotgun Options | 37 |
| Assistive Devices | 39 |
| Shotgun Lesson Plans | 41 |

## 8. Archery Theory & Assistive Devices    51

| | |
|---|---|
| Bows | 51 |
| Assistive Devices | 52 |
| Archery Lesson Plans | 57 |

Appendix I -
*Accessibility Standards*                    67
Appendix II -
*Accessibility Checklist*                    68
Appendix III -
*Hunter Education Administrators*            70
Appendix IV -
*US Fish and Wildlife Service Region Offices*  76
Appendix V -
*National Organizations*                     79
Appendix VI -
*Adaptive Equipment Manufacturers*           83
Appendix VII -
*Publications*                               87
Appendix VIII -
*Often Used Sign Language and Finger Spelling*  90
Glossary -
*Shooting Sports Terms*                      91

# Preface

People throughout the world enjoy a variety of recreational activities. Many of these people share a similar interest and enthusiasm for the rapidly growing recreational activity known as the shooting sports. Educators have the opportunity to develop positive attitudes that will encourage more people, regardless of their abilities, to become active in this wonderful recreational activity.

The purpose of this manual is to provide suggestions on how to structure a class that can be helpful to all students, and ways to use a person's *abilities* to overcome any *disabilities* they may have. Ideas and resources for creating and using adaptive devices when and where they are needed are provided.

This manual will also inform instructors of terminology and techniques that may be new to them. This means taking a close look at shooting sports programs and, case by case, building a system that integrates, rather than segregates.

This manual will start educators on the path towards developing a shooting sports program which is available to anyone wishing to participate. The process is relatively simple for the creative and open-minded instructor. By taking an enthusiastic, imaginative and problem-solving approach, modifications and improvements to programs will achieve this goal.

Making a shooting sports program available to all persons has legal, as well as social and practical, benefits. Programs should assure that every student will receive as close to the same benefits as those received by any other student.

Teaching and leading requires courage, and the willingness to learn and change. Instructors learn by growing and progressing, and change by looking at the past, present and future. This approach will give instructors the tools needed to offer a *complete* shooting sports program to *all* people.

The information contained in this manual is intended to be used in conjunction with an existing program, or as part of a new program, and instructors should feel free to modify, adapt and use any of the teaching tips and lesson plans presented in the manual. The emphasis in this publication, through the use of various examples, is to encourage the generation of ideas and modifications to deal with individual situations.

# Introduction

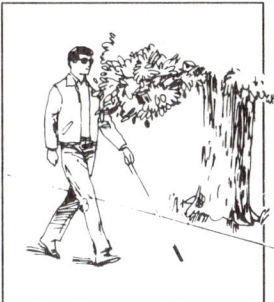

Teachers, instructors and physical health professionals that currently have shooting sports in their programs, or those who are planning to offer it in the future, often feel apprehensive when teaching students with disabilities. Most of that apprehension can be defined as a simple lack of knowledge of the facts.

It is estimated that there are over 43 million persons with disabilities in North America today. That estimate includes persons with varying degrees of mobility limitations, those with mild to severe visual limitations, those with hearing impairments and those with mental and learning impairments. Then, factor in the 10 percent of the population who are age 65 or older, and their incalculable disabilities such as diabetes, arthritis, rheumatism, cardiac and respiratory problems. By combining these various groups, as much as 42 percent of the population has some sort of disability. As the average age of the population increases, so will the percentage of persons with disabilities. A shooting sports program should be designed for **everyone**, rather than just a portion of the population.

# Disability Legislation

There are three United States laws and one Canadian law addressing disability access. The first U.S. law was passed in 1968, and another in 1973. They were amended in 1978 to read; "No otherwise qualified handicapped individual in the United States . . . shall, solely by reason of his handicap, be excluded from the participation in, be denied the benefits of, or be subject to discrimination under any program or activity receiving federal financial assistance."

The latest law, *The Americans with Disabilities Act of 1990*, made it illegal to discriminate against anyone who has a mental or physical disability in the areas of employment, public service, transportation, public accommodations and telecommunications. This act now guarantees that the 43 million citizens with disabilities, have equal opportunity to participate in and contribute to all phases of society. Similarly, the Canadian Charter of Rights states that; "Every individual is equal before and under the law and has the right to the equal protection and equal benefit of the law without discrimination and, in particular, without discrimination based on race, national or ethnic origin, color, religion, sex, age, mental or physical disability." These landmark civil rights laws require that shooting sports programs accommodate all persons regardless of their abilities.

The information contained in this book is intended to be used in conjunction with an existing program or as part of a new program and instructors should feel free to modify, adapt and use any of the teaching tips and lesson plans presented in the book. The emphasis in this publication, through the use of various examples, is to encourage the generation of ideas and modifications to deal with individual situations.

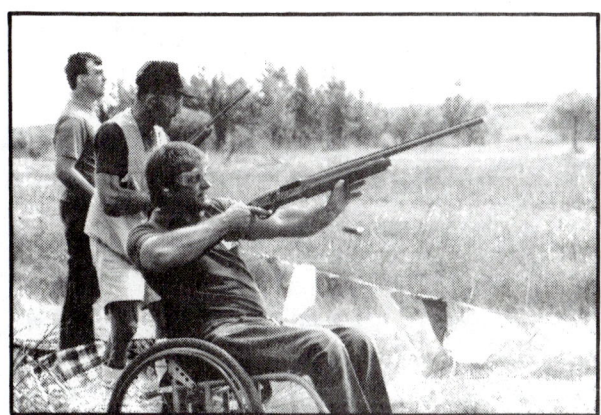

*Outdoor activities are no longer "off-limits" to the physically disabled. In the true spirit of the outdoorsman, they improvise and overcome to enjoy the shooting and hunting sports.*

# 1. Guidelines for Disabilities

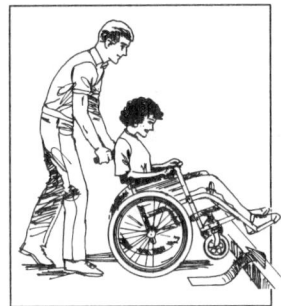

Throughout this manual are terms which may or may not be familiar. Many of the terms that are familiar may now have a different definition. Information is provided in this section to eliminate any distortions, misconceptions, as well as attitudinal barriers, that people with disabilities have faced over the years due to inadequate terminology.

In most personal and social relationships labels are rarely used, except perhaps as a sign of endearment. However, in a legal or professional sense, there is often a need to categorize people to make them eligible for a privilege, such as a student loan, low income housing, or special educational opportunities. In class, approach a student as an individual and a person, rather than someone with a disability.

Words can bring people together, or they can push them apart. The words that have been used interchangeably for many years are "impairment," "disability" and "handicap." Even to this day, many people use them incorrectly, and so distinguishing the differences is important.

Most people have one or several *disabilities*, in one form or another. If someone does not have 20/20 vision, then that person has a disability — less than perfect eyesight. The *handicap* or *impairment* is that vision may be blurred at long range, or there could be difficulty reading small print. When dealing in plain semantics, it should be remembered that disabilities don't always create a handicap or impairment in every situation.

As far as students with impairments, disabilities and handicaps are concerned, teachers must deal with the handicap or impairment the student's disability has created. This can be done through modification of the activity or by modifying the environment in which the activity takes place. One example of this is a person who has blurred vision when looking at a target 60 feet away. This handicap can be addressed with prescription glasses thus modifying the activity, or the environment can be modified by bringing the target closer.

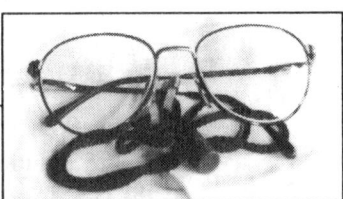

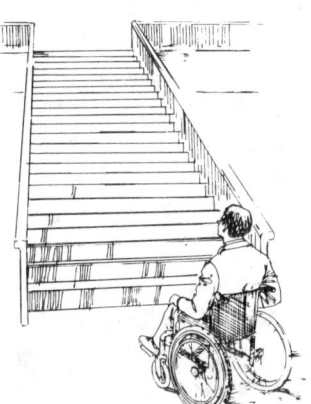

*Ramps or elevators can be added to the facility to eliminate difficulty. The person is assisted past the barrier, or a new, more accessible location can be obtained for the event.*

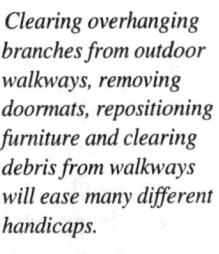

*Narrow doors, poor telephone placement or handles put at levels that are inconsistent with a wheelchair user's needs can create problems.*

*Clearing overhanging branches from outdoor walkways, removing doormats, repositioning furniture and clearing debris from walkways will ease many different handicaps.*

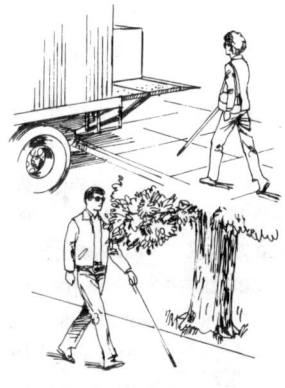

*Another example of a handicap or impairment is the lack of range accessibility, resulting from any of a long list of disabilities. Steps, high curbs, inclines and improperly designed facilities can all create a handicap or impairment.*

The activity of hitting a baseball can be modified by choking up on a bat or getting a longer, heavier or lighter bat, depending on the handicap. How does this apply to a hunting class?

As shown in the above examples, focus should be on the actual handicap to the planned activity and not on the disability causing the handicap. Instructors must make a major effort to dispose of preconceived ideas of which handicaps are associated with a particular disability. In reality, the handicap may only exist in the instructor's mind. Throughout this manual, a realistic look is taken at many disabilities, and the knowledge given to properly appraise a handicap, if it exists, examine it and then resolve it.

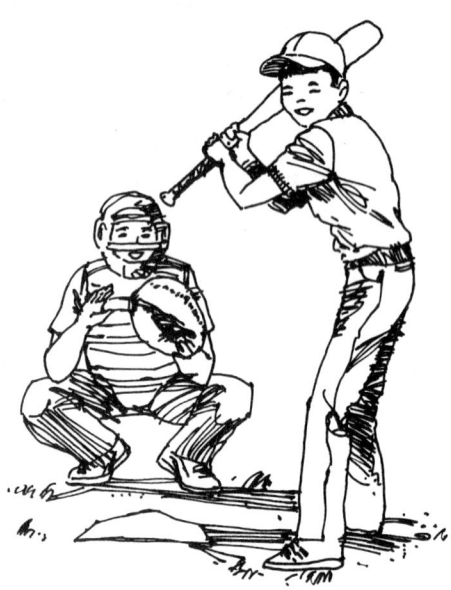

## Physical Impairments

The term "physical impairment" covers many types of physical disabilities and deals with the degree to which the disability has affected the individual. When speaking of a person with a physical disability, talk about specific conditions such as arthritic or rheumatoid disabilities, cerebral palsy, epilepsy, multiple sclerosis, muscular dystrophy, poliomyelitis, spina bifida, spinal cord injuries and paraplegia. Or, speak of conditions that could produce multiple impairments such as a physical impairment in addition to any combination of hearing, visual, mental or learning impairments. The point that must be remembered is, each physical disability will have its own set of handicaps, centering around mobility and strength limitations. In the next chapter, *Disability Awareness*, many of these disabilities, the handicaps they cause and specific ways to resolve the handicaps for the enjoyment of the shooting sports are covered.

## Mental Impairments

Included in this category are two very broad disabilities. Mental illness is a broad description of many psychiatric or emotional states. It is further broken down into "neuroses" which may cause a person to be depressed, anxious or tense to a higher degree than usual, and the rarer "psychosis" which cause delusions, hallucinations and the lack of knowing that the individual's own behavior is abnormal.

The second broad category is mental retardation, which occurs because of damage to the brain. The damage can be the result of a variety of causes such as hormone deficiencies and birth or genetic defects. The degree of the disability, as with all the other impairments, varies enormously and governs the handicap and the modifications needed.

## Learning Impairments

In 1968, learning disabilities received the first official recognition as a separate educational category by the U.S. Department of Education, taking it out of the general mental disability category. Persons with learning disabilities generally have average to above average intelligence, but experience difficulty in one or more basic processes using the spoken or written word. These problems can occur in listening, talking, reading, writing, spelling or math. In many areas of learning disabilities, few if any cause handicaps to the person actively participating in the shooting sports. As a teacher, the main goal will be to identify the particular form the disability has taken, decide if it creates a handicap and proceed from there. An example would be a person with hyperkinetic behavior or "hyperactivity." This behavior affects areas of basic skills because the person can't be still long enough to complete a task. For this person, a highly structured program with clear rules and one activity at a time would be a major part of the modification process.

Misconceptions and myths have always been the major handicap of persons with disabilities. So often, the person's perceived handicap exists only in the teachers' mind, or the minds of other students.

## Hearing Impairments

Hearing disabilities are probably the second most common disability in modern society. As far as shooting sports are concerned, this disability will not cause as many difficulties for the participants as other disabilities might. The main teaching tasks will be to assess the degree of the disability and then adjust methods of communication to resolve any handicap. There are two types of hearing disabilities: one is any of a varying degree of hearing loss. Some form of hearing device to amplify sound is needed. Depending on their hearing loss, the student may still need to watch the instructor's mouth and partially read lips in conjunction with the sounds they are hearing. The other form of hearing disability is deafness, where the person is unable to understand sounds even with amplification. Two-way communication techniques may need to be used such as *signing, lip-reading*, writing or any of the new keyboard devices now available.

## Visual Impairments

Visual disabilities vary from lack of *acuity* (clearness) and *field* (the angle of vision) to *legally blind* and *totally blind*. The degree of the disability is measured against the "20/20" formula. The formula means that in one eye a person can see at 20 feet what a person with the benchmark perfect 20/20 vision can see at 20 feet. An example of a visual disability is if someone has 20/100 in one eye. That means that at 20 feet that eye can only see what a person with perfect vision can see at 100 feet. Visual disabilities can also encompass difficulty in perceiving colors, or an extreme sensitivity or insensitivity to light. The degree of the disability will govern the amount of the handicap and, in turn, the amount of modification needed either to the environment or the activity.

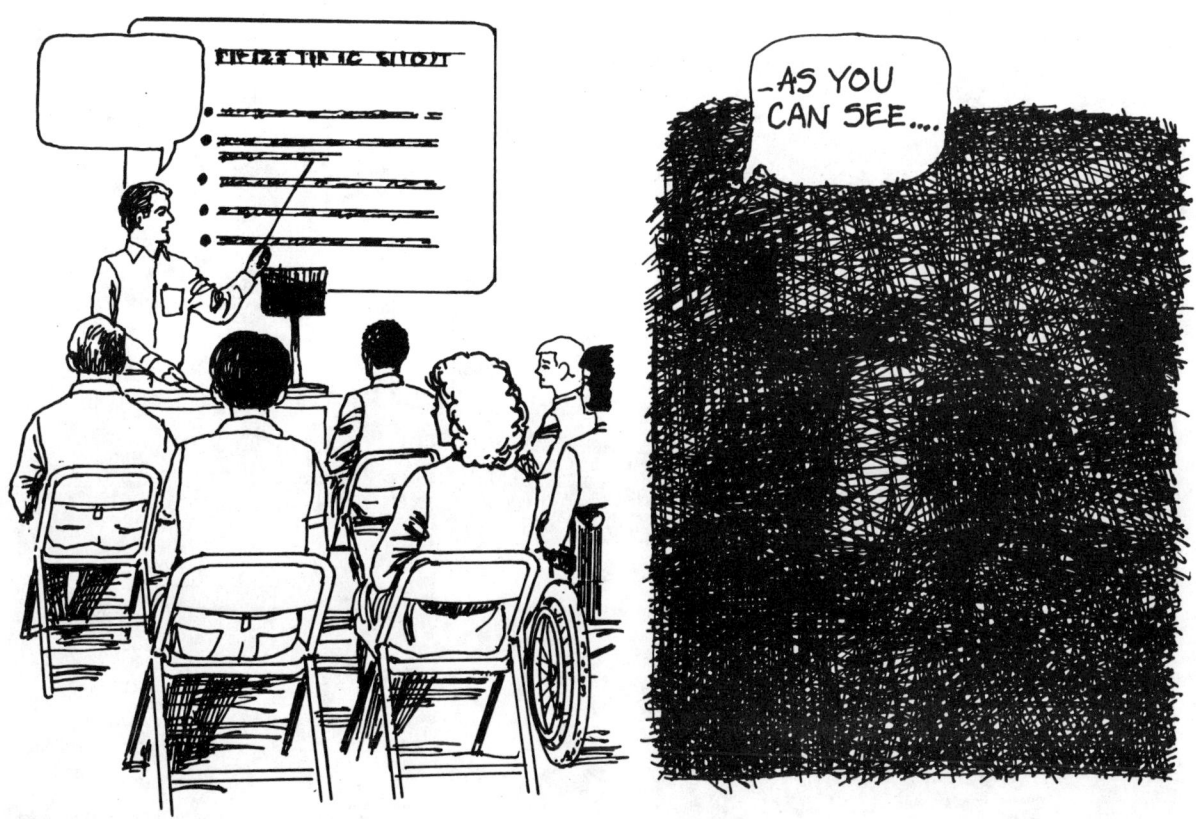

# 2. Disability Awareness

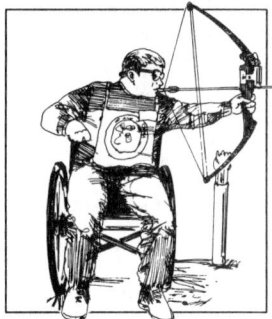

Persons with disabilities have the same needs as every other person in the world. Students need to feel the joy of learning, sharing and growing, and to experience new challenges. No matter what the disability, all persons have the potential to become whatever *they* want to be. It is not an instructor's job to attempt to regulate what the person can or cannot accomplish.

**Communication:** An instructor's major concern is communication with students. Addressing the impairments or handicaps that some disabilities cause may require modification of communications techniques. Deal with the person, not the disability. Treat adults as adults, and not as children. Talk to the person with the disability and not just to the companion who may be along with them. When offering help, wait until they accept it, as they are the only ones who really know if they need help or not. Take cues from the person with the disability concerning what they can or cannot do, and don't emphasize any supposed differences in their abilities.

There are a variety of impairments or handicaps, and many ways and levels to communicate with the individual students that address their impairments yet still allow them to feel they are part of the group.

## Students with Physical Impairments

Because there is such a wide range of causes, definitions, and severities of physical disabilities, there is no recognized system for classifying a disability by degree. Terms referring to physical conditions such as "paraplegia," "cerebral palsy" and "muscular dystrophy" are good clinical descriptions but have little functional meaning, since people with the same condition differ greatly in what they can do. The best way to determine what a person can do or not do is to ask them.

Knowing the abilities of the student is very important. Keep in mind that individuals with the same physical condition will vary in both preferences and abilities to do the same task.

Thousands of people have some degree of physical disability. Just because they have disabilities does not mean they can't do everything required in a shooting sports class.

Mobility poses the biggest problem for many students. Fortunately, shooting doesn't require a great deal of movement. In situations requiring movement, (swinging a shotgun for example) throwing targets straight away from the shooter, instead of at an angle, can help some students succeed.

Lack of strength poses a problem for some persons with disabilities. Equipment such as the tripod gun rest can alleviate the problem in many cases, as can a lighter weight, smaller-calibered firearm.

### When working with people with physical disabilities:

Don't assume that a person in a wheelchair needs help. If the person requests help, by all means help, but don't assume they *want* it. If a person with a disability falls, wait for them to say that they need help getting up before helping them to their feet.

Be patient without being protective or overindulgent. Although a person may not be progressing as fast as the rest of the class, it may be very important to them to do it *themselves*.

Crutches, canes, and wheelchairs are necessary pieces of equipment. Do not put them in the closet or roll them out of the way to "tidy up." Doing so leaves their owner stranded.

Allow all students to do all the activities offered. Do not underestimate the capabilities or interests of the individual.

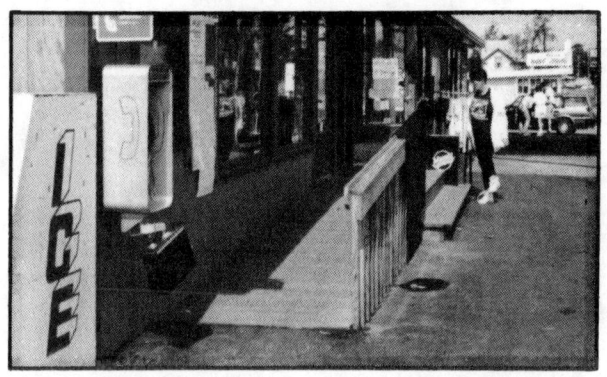

**Personal aids and devices:**

People with physical disabilities often depend on tools to increase their functional abilities. Typically, those tools such as a wheelchair loading device on the top of their car, or a custom made, ultra-lite racing wheelchair, become as personal to that person as clothes do to others. As a result, any handling of a person's tools should be done carefully and considerately.

In most situations, the person has complete mastery of their equipment and will not need help with it. If they do need help it is not only proper, but usually necessary, to ask them how to help. For children, ask a parent or guardian how to assist them.

Some pieces of equipment have rules or restrictions regarding what the operator can do while using them. Ask the user what might cause trouble, i.e. vibration, shock, or extremes of temperature.

## Students with Hearing Impairments

Hearing impairments are among the most common of disabilities. As with other disabilities, there are different levels of hearing impairment. People who are "hard of hearing" have difficulty hearing other people's speech, but can understand it with the help of amplification. People who are "deaf" cannot hear sound well enough to distinguish it, even with amplification.

A person who is hearing impaired may also have trouble speaking clearly, since he/she may not be able to hear well enough to correct pronunciation errors in their own speech. People tend to speak the way they hear. Some people with severe hearing impairments may choose not to use their voices.

"Lip-reading" is a technique learned by some people with hearing impairments. It assists them in understanding the speech of others. Lip-readers watch a speaker's mouth and identify words by the shape and position of the lips and tongue. This is a difficult skill to master, since less than 35 percent of English words are recognizable solely by mouth positions and movements. Do not expect your hearing-impaired students to read lips. Body language and what the speaker is saying are very important.

Signing and writing are often used by people with speech impairments as well as hearing impairments. For some, writing is the only means of communication available. People with hearing or speech impairments generally find communication to be their main problem, rather than the techniques of a particular activity.

Interpreters who translate verbal language into sign language are often necessary in order to include people with severe hearing impairments. Often, finding an interpreter can be accomplished by checking with the student's family to locate a volunteer. Ask other people with hearing impairments for a reference, or call the local department of rehabilitation or social services for suggestions. Check with special education personnel in the school system for interpreters who are teachers or aides. Contact local technical or community colleges for names of instructors who teach sign language, and check the community service listings in the phone book for agencies that serve people with hearing impairments.

**When working with people
who have hearing impairments:**

If a person appears to need assistance, offer help, but don't give it unless the offer is accepted. Speak directly to the person with the hearing impairment, not to their interpreter, and speak clearly and distinctly at a normal rate and volume. Don't exaggerate the volume or speed of your speech unless you are asked to, and above all be expressive. Use facial expressions, hand gestures and body movements to accentuate speech. Subtle changes in tone or volume to indicate meaning may be missed by someone with a hearing impairment. The more visual clues used, the easier it will be for students to understand. When giving instructions or explanations, keep background noise to a minimum. If it's very loud, go someplace quieter, or give instructions before entering a noisy area. Learn to face people with hearing impairments while speaking. Be sure the instructor's face and upper body are visible, and that he/she is standing close enough to be seen plainly. Avoid shadows on the face caused by broad-rimmed hats or sunglasses. Try to avoid eating, smoking, or chewing while talking. It makes speech much harder to understand. Be sure to have the attention of the person spoken to before starting, perhaps by touching their arm. It is important that they understand one topic before going on to the next. Do not be afraid to repeat instructions if there is confusion — perhaps rephrase the statement. Use visual aids in addition to verbal instructions to create better understanding. Incorporating visual cues in directions and instructions, such as a hot/cold indicator flag or light on the range, will make the environment all the more accessible.

# Students with Visual Impairments

People describe vision quality (or the lack of) in terms of acuity (clearness) and field of view (the angle or width of what the eyes can see). However, it is important to remember that there are vision problems that affect people in ways other than clarity and field of view. Color blindness and extreme sensitivity to light are two typical examples.

People with visual impairments get different amounts of visual information from their surroundings. It is important to realize that while vision does provide people with a great deal of information about their environment, it is not the only source.

People with visual impairments frequently learn to rely on other senses to fill in the gaps created by their limited ability to see. Senses such as smell, touch, hearing and the perception of movement, all become more important.

This increased dependence on the other senses is a key element in making activities accessible to a person who has impaired vision. This usually means taking advantage of the abilities they have developed, in order to compensate for their inability to see clearly.

The only way to definitely know how much a person can or cannot see is to ask them. Don't make assumptions. Be imaginative when assisting people with visual disabilities; find ways to deal with the resulting impairments.

## When working with people with visual impairments:

If someone seems to need assistance, offer help but don't give it unless the offer is accepted. If it is accepted, ask for an exact explanation of how to help. Generally, a vision impairment has no affect on a person's hearing or their mental abilities, so don't shout at, or talk down to, a person with a visual impairment. Talk directly to them and not to others on their behalf. Don't be afraid to use words such as "see," "look" or "blind." Such words are part of everyday vocabulary, and persons with a visual impairment use them, too. When meeting a person who is blind, be sure to identify yourself and remember to let them know when leaving. **Do not pet guide dogs**, especially without the owner's permission. A dog in a harness is on duty, and if the dog is distracted the owner may be placed in jeopardy.

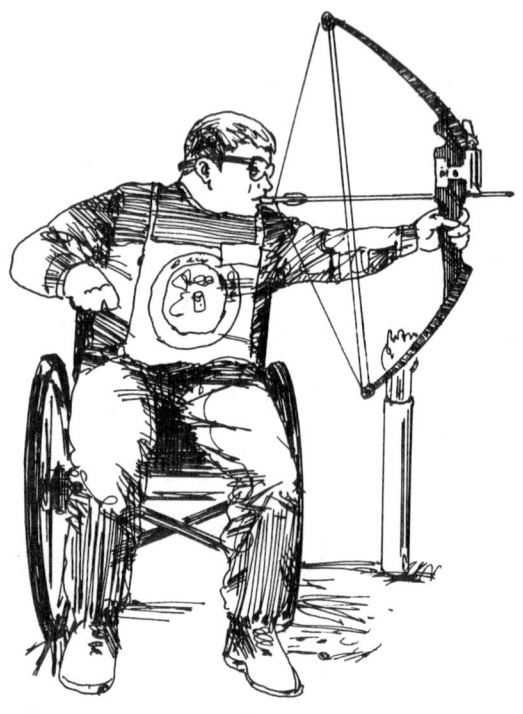

Use specific, descriptive language when giving directions. Use colors, textures, movements, and directional indicators to make directions more vivid for the person with a visual impairment. Orient the person with the visual impairment to the placement of objects around them. The analogy of using the clock face to pinpoint locations works well for all people, not just those with disabilities. For example: "The bottle of cleaning oil is at nine o'clock, and the patches are at three o'clock, on your table." When seating a person who has a visual disability, place their hand on the back of the seat and let them seat themselves. Orient the person to new environments by describing sizes, shapes, distances, and any obstacles or hazards. Minimize noise — high levels of background noise can be very distracting and confusing to a person who relies on their hearing for information about their surroundings. When demonstrating a skill, the person with a visual impairment may want to hold the instructor's hands as they work. Explain graphically, in concrete terms, what is being done as it is done. Sometimes it's best to stand behind a person and reach through their arms, so they can follow the exact movements of the instructor.

## When assisting someone with a visual impairment:

If someone with poor vision accepts an offer to guide them, ask "Would you like to take my arm?" Brush a forearm against theirs so the blind person can grip the arm above the elbow. Children will grip the same way, only at the wrist. Some aged and/or disabled will want to walk arm-in-arm because it offers more support. *Important! Don't attempt to lead someone by taking his or her arm!*

The instructor's arm should be relaxed at their side, while the person's arm will be bent at the elbow. The instructor should keep the student's arm close to their body.

While using the sighted guide method, the person with the visual impairment should walk half a step behind the guide. The guide must walk at that person's pace. If the person being guided pulls back or tightens their grip, the guide is probably going too fast. Never try to push or steer any person in front, and always remember to mention ramps, stairs, narrow hallways, doors, etc. Add whether the stairs go up or down, which way the door opens, and when they've reached the last step.

**When opening doors:**

When approaching a door, say so. Keep the person's free-hand side to the door. Tell them which way the door opens and allow the person to hold the door open.

## Students with Mental Impairments

The terms "mental retardation" and "mental handicap" are now outdated. Instructor's must refer to students with a slower ability to learn as "developmentally disabled." There are different levels or categories of developmental disability. The general categories used are mild, moderate, severe, and profound. The range between mild and severe is extremely broad. Many people who are developmentally disabled can easily participate in shooting classes.

People who are developmentally disabled may also have accompanying physical disabilities, and may require help with some tasks. Be sure to consider if they will need help to participate in an activity. If so, make sure that an instructor, a friend, or a volunteer understands how to provide that assistance.

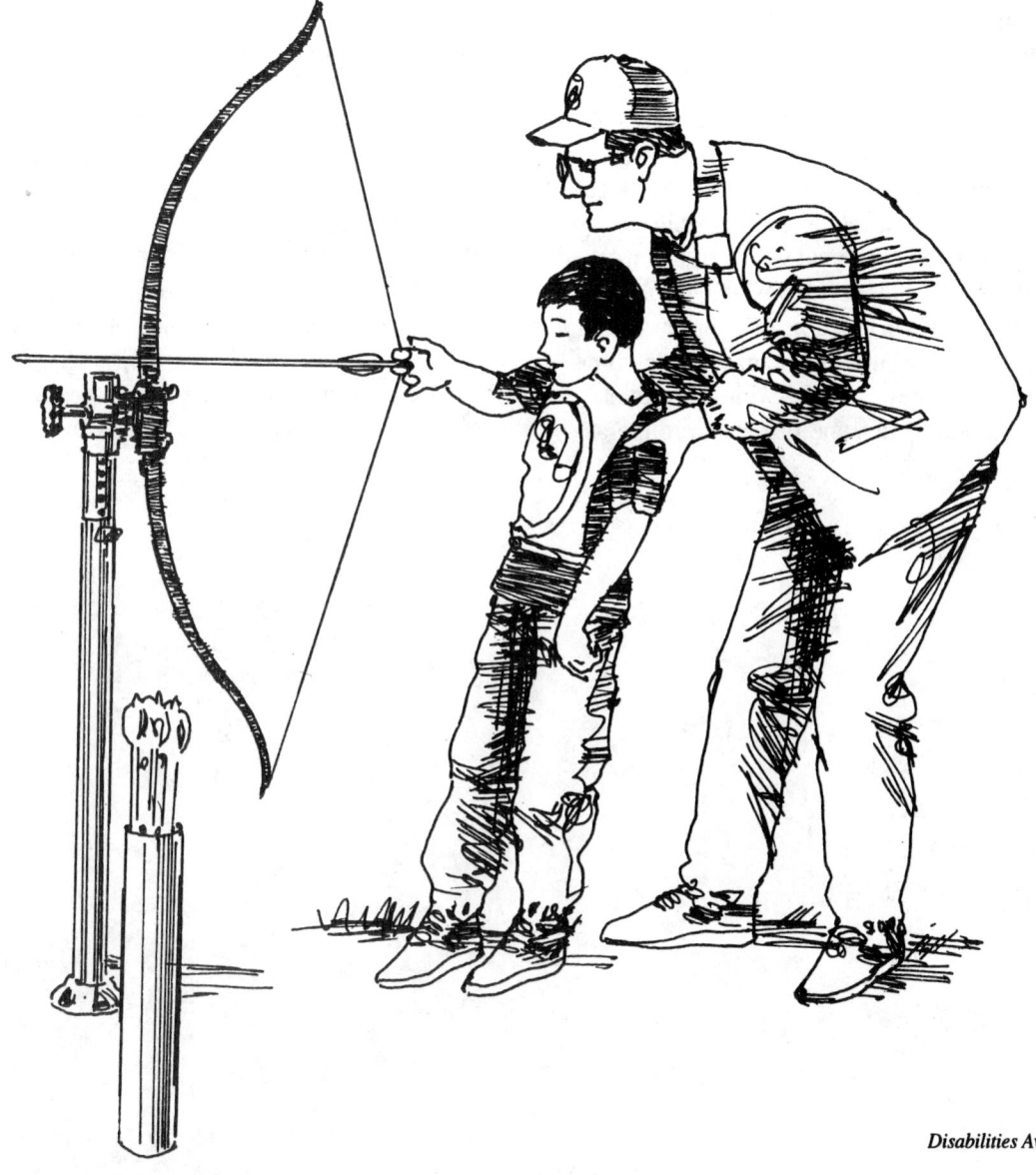

Disabilities Awareness 11

**When working with students
who are developmentally disabled:**

Concentrate on the abilities and interests of each individual and don't underestimate those abilities or interests. Break down directions into small steps that can be learned sequentially, and demonstrate where possible. Speak to students with dignity and respect, regardless of their learning ability level. Keep in mind that some people's ability to *understand* speech is much better developed than their ability to *create* speech. Don't talk about a person in front of them, a speech problem does not mean they can't understand. Provide positive feedback for positive experiences, not negative feedback for negative experiences. If the person appears to need help, wait until the offer to help is accepted. It may be very important for them to do something *themselves* even if they don't do it perfectly.

The structure of the activities is important. If a short attention span is a problem, provide a variety of activities with different tasks. Allow plenty of time for learning and completion of a task and, above all, repetition is extremely important.

Before beginning a new activity, review the safety rules. A person with a developmental disability may lack the judgement to understand which situations are dangerous. Persons with developmental disabilities may not be aware of what action is inappropriate or appropriate, so discuss it with them. Provide some non-competitive games and activities, preferably ones that don't eliminate some players from the action.

# Students with Learning Impairments

People with learning disabilities often have average to above average intelligence. However, they lack a particular skill to complete the learning process. Learning disabilities take many forms and may involve any of an individual's senses.

- Some read "saw" for "was" and write "71" for "17."
- Some have difficulty with sequential things like yesterday, today, and tomorrow.
- Some cannot remember well.
- Many have difficulty with specific sources of information. For example, auditory learners retain spoken information well but have great difficulty retaining information they read.
- Some have poor coordination or timing.

**In order to facilitate learning:**

- Use a variety of formats (verbal, visual, and physical) to communicate information.
- Break down skills into smaller parts.
- Use colors or symbols to differentiate left from right, front from back, etc.

People with what are called "behavior-motor functioning difficulties" may be over-active, behave impulsively, or have coordination problems. When instructing, provide clearly defined activity spaces (range, classroom). Complete one activity before starting another, and provide a variety of activities so that everyone's strengths will shine through.

# 3. Access for All People

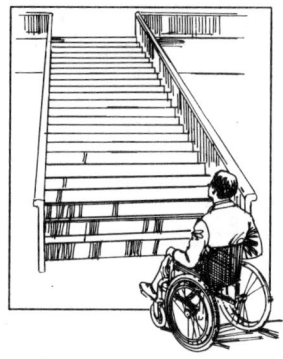

The Americans with Disabilities Act of 1990 has mandated access to all people, but in reality, complete access at every facility will take time. During this implementation period, flexibility will be important in planning programs and finding facilities at which to hold classes. **Endeavor only to use facilities that are fully accessible to all students**. The following is information that, even if as a last resort, will help utilize facilities that have not been made fully accessible.

## Wheelchair Pointers

**Moving a wheelchair:**
- Don't lift or steer with the armrests, as they come off.
- Don't let fingers get between the seat and the frame because they could be crushed.
- When lifting, grab the frame, not the wheels.

**Taking a wheelchair up stairs:**
- This is a two-person job!
- Position the chair against the bottom step, back to the stairs.
- Standing on the first step, take a firm grip and lift the chair onto the first step.
- The second person must stand below the chair to lift and steady the chair as it goes up the stairs. They must hold the frame, not the wheels.
- Make sure the second person is strong enough to hold the weight of the chair and its occupant in case it slips.

**Carrying a wheelchair down stairs:**
- This is a two-person job!
- Do not attempt to take an occupied wheelchair down stairs unless the occupant's weight and the weight of the chair can be lifted repeatedly, and full control can be maintained.
- Grasp the handgrips and tip the chair back. With the second person holding the chair from below, slowly move the chair forward to the stairs.
- The lifters must use their bodies as a brake starting at the first step. Don't wait until the chair falls to do so.
- Rest between steps.

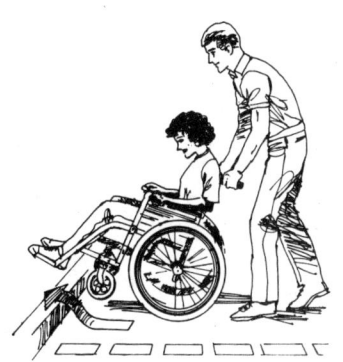

**Pushing a wheelchair up a curb:**
- Tip the chair back and place the front wheels on top of the curb.
- Lift/push the chair onto the curb.

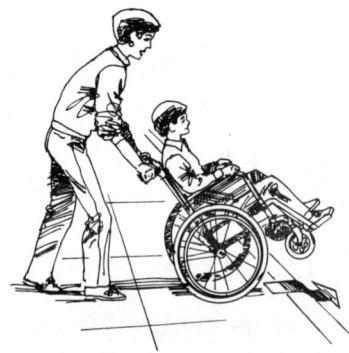

**Pushing a wheelchair down a curb:**
- Place your foot on the tipping lever. Take firm hold of the handgrips, then tip the chair backward.
- Gently lower the chair down the curb, taking some of the weight yourself and making sure both wheels hit the ground at the same time.

*Instructor's note: The publisher does not recommend these pointers. They have been included only for the person who wishes to take the responsibility for moving a wheelchair.*

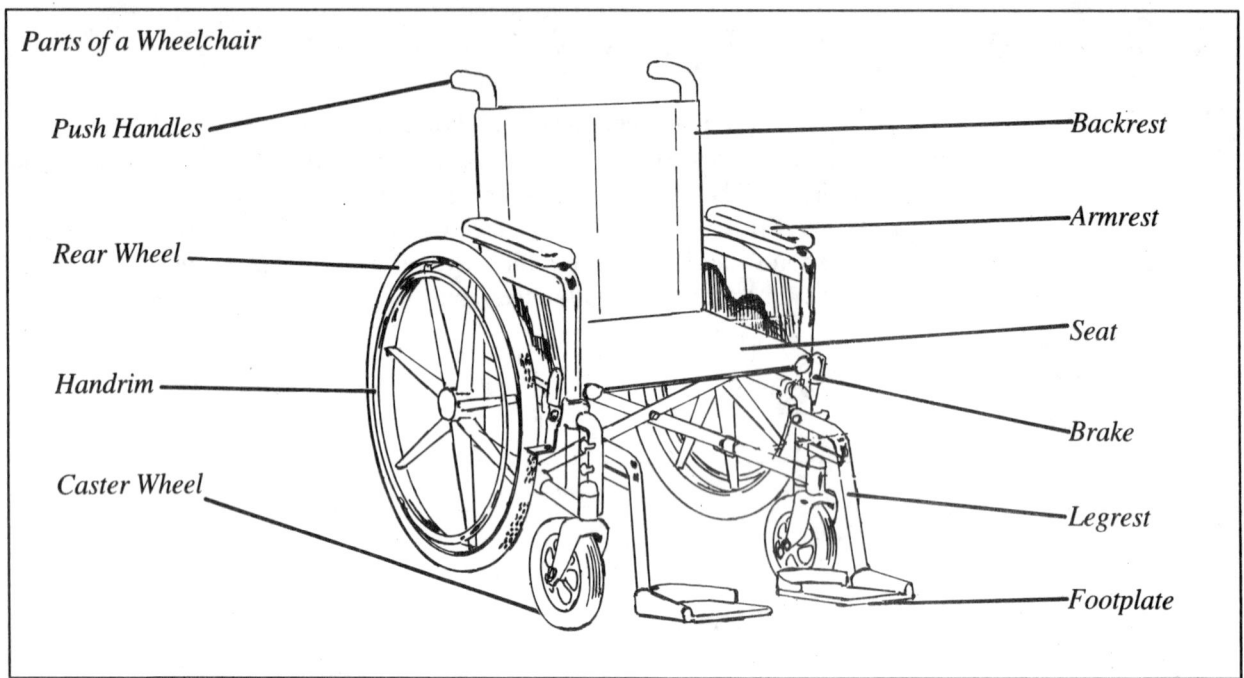

*Parts of a Wheelchair*

## Change of Environment

A change in the program's environment can accomplish several major goals. It can provide access to certain individuals, it can eliminate a handicap and it can make the activity more enjoyable for all participants. The one idea that educators must constantly reinforce is — don't create access for one person that will turn into a handicap for another. An example would be if a "guideline" for a person with a visual impairment was improperly placed on the shooting range, making it a barrier for a person with a physical impairment. An example of a proper change is a ramp — an environmental change that can benefit persons with physical impairments and the elderly, without impairing other students. Railings on the ramp can aid students with visual impairments. Directional beepers that are activated on the shooting line are a direct benefit to the shooter with a visual impairment, and adding a target that shows a hit (balloons, exploding targets, etc.) is of benefit to the shooter with a hearing impairment. In all these cases, the bottom line is that the change in the environment must not handicap any other shooters.

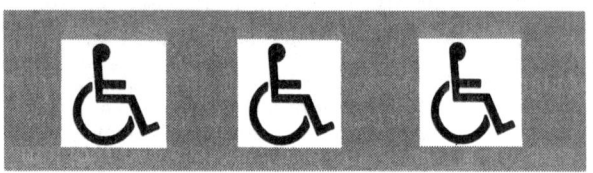

## Change the Program

All people learn differently. Instructors must learn to recognize the different learning styles of students and either modify methods or bring additional teachers in to address different students. Some students may need total "hands-on" learning experiences, or do better with written directions. Others may be very productive using spoken or visual directions. An instructor, teaching to any group of students using only one style, will only reach part of the class.

Program changes can run from various forms of special scoring systems to the use of adaptive devices. An example is the "Spot Round" for archery competition. Students shoot two complete rounds at a 40 cm target from 20 yards. By referring to a handicap chart, students are then switched to the proper-sized target to fit their skill level. From that point on, the students compete on equal levels with periodic adjustments for improvement in their skill level.

Another example of a program change is once again to add a balloon to the center of the target to provide either a visual or auditory alert of a hit. Imagination, modification and communication are the key elements to bring a shooting sports program into the mainstream, and allow all people to learn and enjoy. To be flexable enough to modify the program or the product where needed and to be able to communicate your needs and understand the needs of others is the goal of both the teacher and the student.

*14  Access for All People*

# 4. Instructor and Student Safety

No matter what is done to promote safety, teaching the shooting sports will always hold a certain element of danger. Instructors have given their ideas on how to make the profession a safer one for those on the firing line.

Close adherence to range procedure is, of course, the best way to avoid problems with safety. However, there are a few things instructors can do to protect themselves, their students and keep problems from happening.

## Range Procedure Tips

By dividing the range space into shooting and non-shooting areas, only instructors and the students they are working with are allowed to get close to the firing line. This keeps people from wandering close to the shooters, distracting them, and potentially having a safety problem.

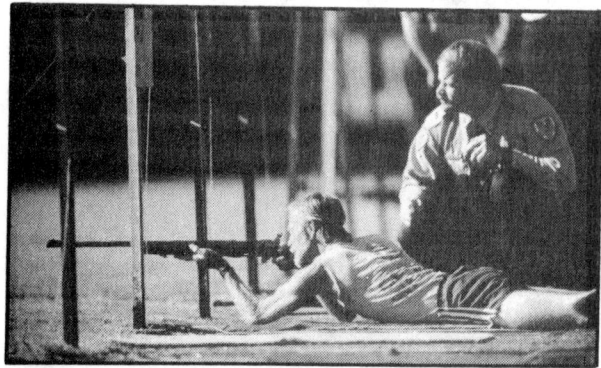

*Shooters with physical disabilities can still participate in shooting competitions and succeed.*

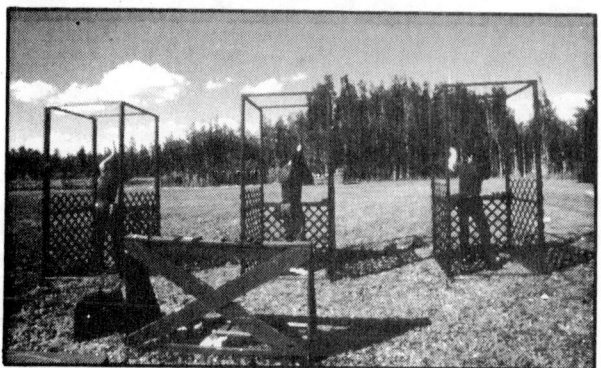

*As these shooters demonstrate, always keep firearms pointed in a safe direction.*

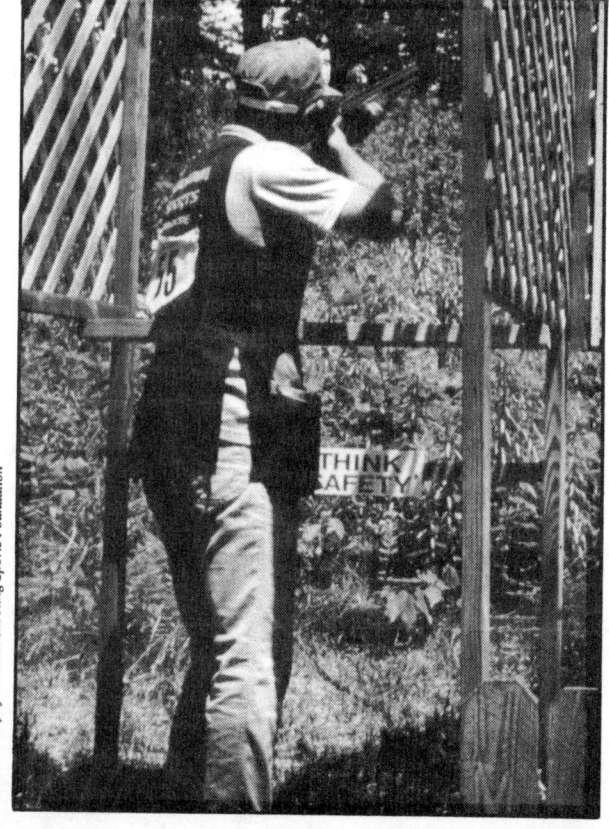

*Photos courtesy of National Shooting Sports Foundation*

Placing a physical barrier, such as a post, between the different shooting lanes not only discourages movement on the part of the shooter, but restrains the shooter's field of fire by limiting his ability to swing the gun from side to side. Similarly, posts on either side of a shotgun shooting box will stop someone from following a target into a dangerous area. Portable doorways can be configured inexpensively from PVC pipes.

Stand close! As the picture shows, if the instructor stands close enough to the student inside the arc of

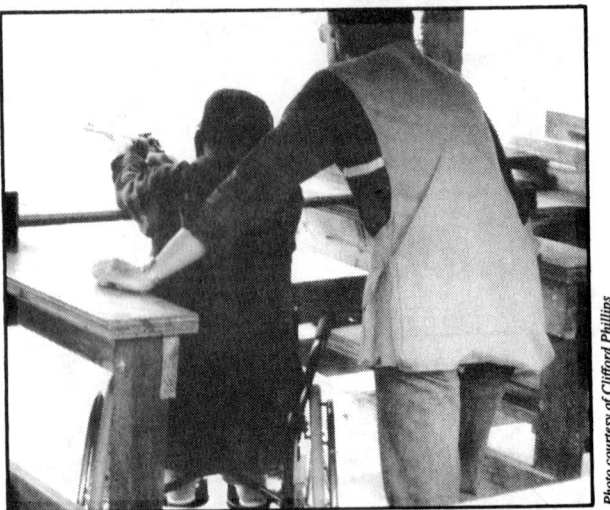

*Shooting positions for the game of Sporting Clays are designed to focus shooter's attention on a specific field of fire.*

the barrel, it's more difficult for the student to accidentally point the gun at the instructor. If the instructor stands behind the student, the student's elbows and shoulders are easier to reach, and the barrel must travel further to point at the instructor.

If the student does start to come around with the gun, place a hand against their elbow or shoulder to prevent further swinging. If necessary, the barrel can be blocked if the student's arm doesn't present itself, or you are too far away.

Keeping the student/instructor ratio one to one when live firing gives instructors more control of the line. It is best to have a teacher or helper for each student with a disability. An instructor can't be in two places at once, much less three or four.

One point to consider is that many of the students with disabilities will have an interested parent or friend who will bring them to the class. Don't have them just watch the class — have them take the class as a student. This will provide one more trained student, it will give the person with the disability a qualified person to shoot with away from the class, and there will be one more student helper.

Avoid shouting at, or taking a gun away from, anyone. If a student out of arm's reach *starts* to come around with the barrel, a shout to them might be appropriate. But if the student already has the gun pointed up-range, shouting at them may only confuse and terrify them as they try to do the right thing — with potentially disastrous results. The same applies to taking a gun from a student in a dangerous situation. When someone, anyone, tries to take something away from another, the immediate reaction is to try to keep it. Talk the student out of the situation in a calm, firm voice and discuss what they did wrong once the situation is resolved.

Don't grab the student, or block his/her swing below the elbow. Grabbing a student may startle them and cause them to tense up — potentially pulling the trigger accidentally. Blocking the student below the elbow can cause the same thing to happen by jarring his/her shooting hand. Stand close and stay calm, and you will assure students of a safe, educational and pleasant experience.

## Program Safety

The safety of all students in the program begins right in the classroom. By ingraining firearm safety into the students' minds, no one in the class should ever have to worry about another person's firearm. Safe firearm handling is when every shooter knows 100 percent of the time what the status of their firearm is. As an instructor, teach through example. A positive attitude, and total control over the class at all times, will teach the students the same attitude toward total control of their firearm.

## Environmental Safety

Many facilities have been made barrier free, while others are still in the process of becoming accessible to all persons with disabilities. It is the class provider's responsibility to determine if barriers still exist in the class facility or if the accessability changes that have been made lend themselves to the shooting sports. It can be little things that are not only irritating, but can pose a real danger (i.e., positioning tables too close for wheelchairs, walkers or crutches, or doormats that cause problems for wheelchairs and crutches and others). As people with disabilities are trained and graduate, they can act as critics on access and safety, and can give helpful suggestions.

*Photo courtesy of Clifford Phillips*

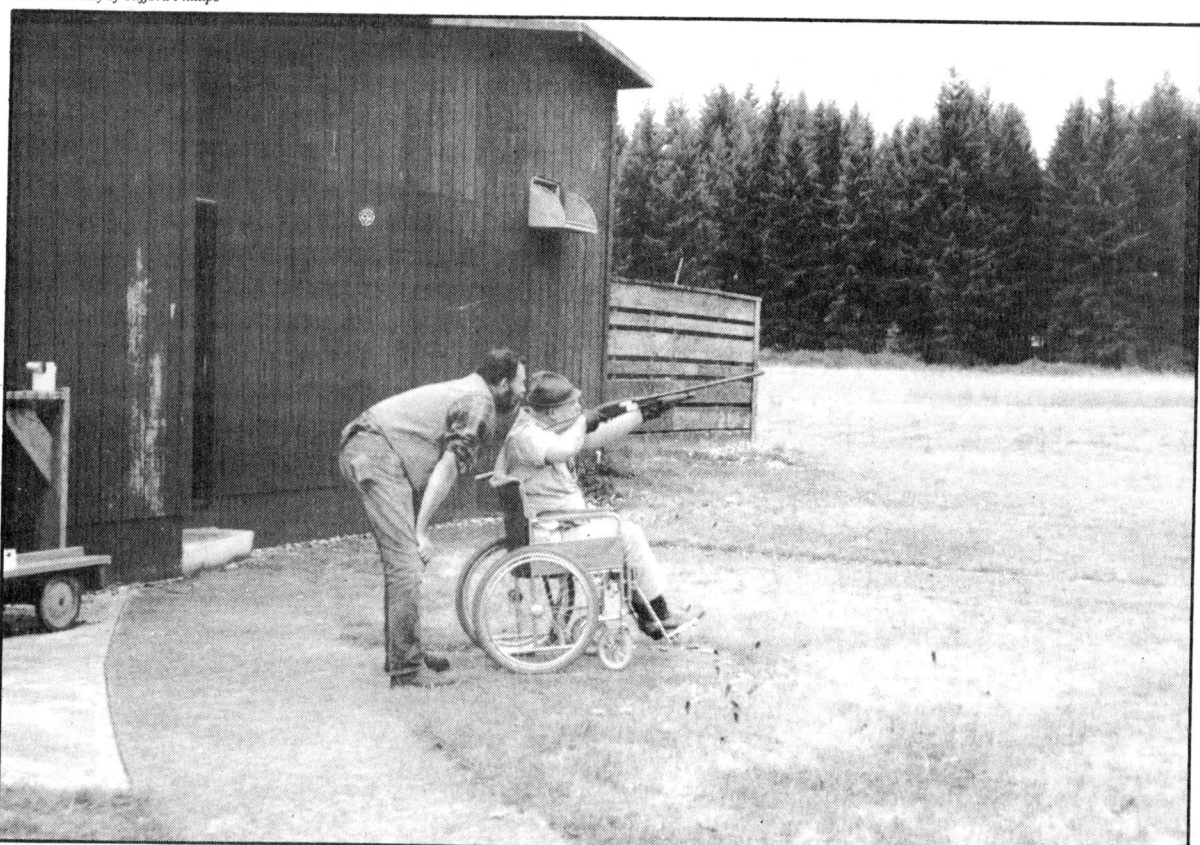

*The attentive instructor will always be in a position where he/she can be of immediate assistance to a new shooter.*

*Instructor and Student Safety* 17

# 5. Teaching Students with Disabilities

Teaching a planned, well-rounded class requires pre-registration of at least two weeks in advance. Identify students' abilities as well as their disabilities and plan to accommodate the group. The goal is to meet individual student's needs.

Students with disabilities may require additional class time and have special needs like space for a wheelchair, or an interpreter who knows sign language. Plan for those needs before the class begins, and try to be prepared for student disabilities which were not discovered at pre-registration. Once the first class has been conducted, the planning stage will be easier. Include people with disabilities in any advertising for the class.

Alternative teaching methods may or may not be needed. Take charge of the group and the environment. Students with multiple disabilities may require more than one adaptive device or approach. Experiment with different teaching methods.

## Some Tips

The following suggestions have been field-tested and work extremely well while teaching students with disabilities:

1. Identify the students' abilities rather than their disabilities. Try not to under or overestimate what the students can do. Different students will need different kinds of help. Talk to the students, or to their parents, teachers, care workers, etc. to better understand the students' abilities and what assistance they might need.
2. Remember that *patience plus persistence equals progress* for all students.
3. Be creative, modify equipment and procedures to allow the students to reach their highest level of performance.
4. Build each lesson plan on previously learned knowledge.
5. Use a variety of teaching methods in classes. Alternate between lectures and practical exercises and use visual aids to play to each student's strengths. Always remember that different students learn differently.
6. Repeat safety rules, fundamentals, and other information frequently.
7. Encourage students to do things independently using as little adaptive equipment as possible.
8. Assist minimally, but whenever necessary.
9. Provide regular feedback whenever something goes right, regardless of the level of success.
10. Use discreet physical contact to correct positions, and to help point the firearm.

# Hunting Opportunities for People with Disabilities

In several jurisdictions, unique hunting opportunities are available to hunters with disabilities. In a recent survey, many state and provincial Fish and Game administrators said that their jurisdictions offered additional hunting opportunities to hunters with disabilities. Typically, people who qualify as "disabled" (the specifications vary) may be able to receive free hunting licenses, permits to hunt from stationary motor vehicles, and permits that allow them to use crossbows. Different jurisdictions have different regulations, but the vast majority have some legislation that pertains to hunters with disabilities. (For more specific information contact the Hunter Education administrators listed in the Appendix.)

On the national level, the United States Fish and Wildlife Service is building accessible hunting blinds throughout the country. Many of these blinds will be placed in national wildlife refuges offering some of the most sought-after hunting opportunities in North America to hunters with disabilities. Guides are now offering opportunities for big game hunting for persons with disabilities, such as using ATVs or snowmobiles to give access to the back country. Many people previously confined to wheelchairs are now going anywhere. Guides are building blinds to accommodate the ATVs, snowmobiles or wheelchairs, and treestands large enough for a wheelchair equipped with an automatic lift. Communities in high recreational areas are beginning to encourage and accomodate sports enthusiasts with disabilities.

To find out about accessible public hunting areas, contact your nearest U.S. and Canadian Fish and Wildlife regional office. A list of the regional offices and their addresses appears in the Appendix.

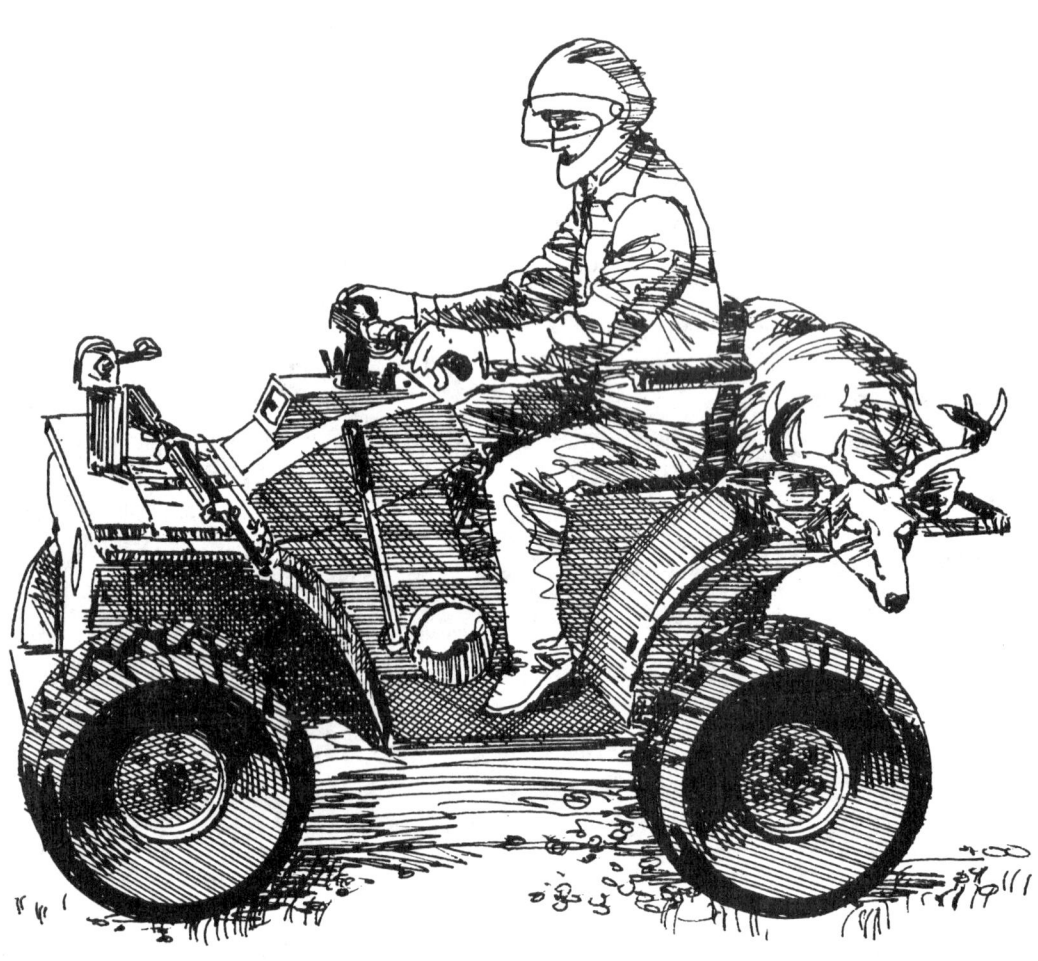

# 6. Rifle/Airgun Theory & Assistive Devices

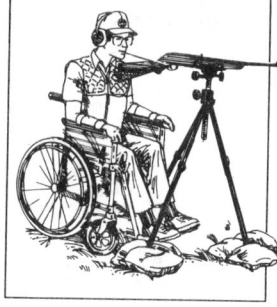

## Theory

One of the most effective ways to teach beginning shooters safety and control is with an airgun. There is virtually no recoil, they help students overcome flinching, while learning trigger and breath control. A competent instructor can use an airgun to teach all the fundamental rules of safe gun handling and marksmanship. The airgun also makes it possible for instructors to teach indoors, as just about any teaching facility, from a classroom to a garage, can safely accomodate an indoor airgun range.

## Airguns

Because of the low recoil and small degree of physical movement involved, airgun target shooting with a rifle or pistol is appropriate for most persons with disabilities. Sportspersons with disabilities can easily compete, and in some cases dominate, airgun target shooting events.

Competitive airgun shooting, as with many other sports, is "gadgety" and technology driven. The skills of the user are crucial, but shooters place great emphasis on creating the best system of assistive devices possible. Most formal events take place at indoor ranges or at paved, covered outdoor ranges as do most informal practices. Commercial, public and club ranges give shooters with disabilities a wide range of shooting opportunities.

Shooting airguns, rather than cartridge-based arms, is a growing trend in the shooting world. Thanks to the limited range of a pellet, lack of noise and the extreme accuracy of modern airguns, airgun ranges are much easier to construct (and keep operating with less public opposition) than even their .22 caliber counterparts. A room with 40 feet of unobstructed space can easily house a regulation airgun range, while as little as 20 feet can house a practice range. Many basements can be converted to a home practice range and many towns have no local ordinances against airgun use within their city limits. In Europe, airgun shooting and competition has become the central focus for many towns. They center their activities around the elaborate shooting centers which in the rural areas become the town's center of activity. By way of comparison, European airgun shooting holds the same status as golf does in the United States.

Quality competition airguns are as accurate as many cartridge-based firearms and cost a great deal less to shoot. Pneumatic and spring-air models run from inexpensive ($50-$100) to very expensive ($1,000-$2,000), but they do require the strength and mobility to cock them in order to fire. However, CO2

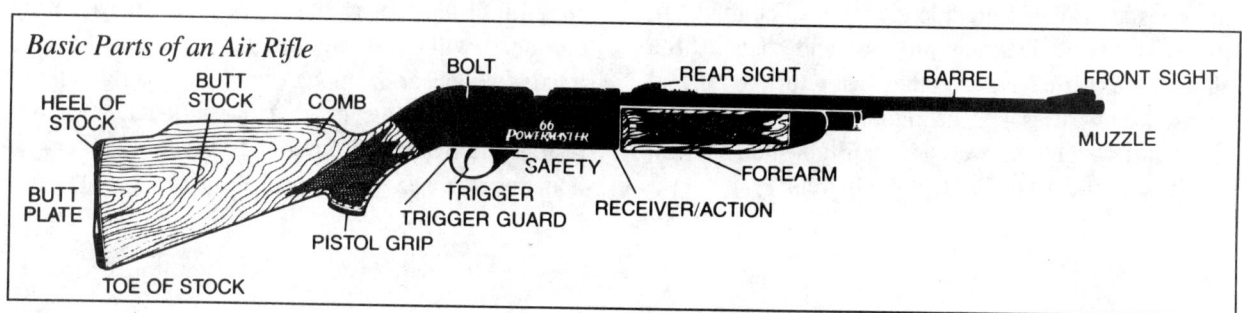

*Basic Parts of an Air Rifle*

models require very few motor skills to shoot, and also come in expensive or inexpensive models. Options run from specialized stock configurations and precision sights to adjustable triggers. Most airgun shooters find that the cost of ammunition is perhaps one-fifth of what .22 target ammunition would cost to shoot.

Many highpower rifle, pistol, trap and skeet shooting coaches are now using airguns as training aids for their students. A firearm's mass weight can be duplicated and in many cases even the recoil of a firearm can be duplicated with a customized airgun. In addition to the lower ammunition cost, airguns make a great training tool because they make extensive practice possible. And, because of the low discharge noise and its flinch-free nature, an airgun lets the shooter learn good habits. Airguns are just beginning to approach velocities of 1,500 feet per second (fps), and those that are used indoors are in the 700 fps range. When compared to a .22 caliber firearm at 1,100-plus fps, the pellet will leave the firearm at a slower speed, causing magnification of any errors on the part of the shooter. However, due to the airgun's negligible recoil and higher degree of safety, both novice shooters and experts can easily learn (or re-learn) the fundamentals of shooting.

## Small Bore and Large Bore Rifle and Pistol

Most small and large bore rifles are available and adaptable to the majority of persons with disabilities. Their mass weight is more than most airguns and their recoil is stronger. But, with proper training and adaptive devices to accommodate the increased power, hunting-sized firearms are not out of the question for the person with disabilities. If access to reloading facilities is available, light loads can also be made up to assist in the learning process, and then as the shooter's experience grows they can return to normal loads. Many rifles and handguns come in standard sizes and weights as well as ultra-light models with composite stocks and lightweight barrels.

## Assistive Devices

Years of research into assistive devices has yielded quite a quantity of products that work well for shooters with disabilities.

### Scopes

Probably the most common assistive device, scopes for both rifles and pistols are available across North America. For shooters with visual disabilities, a large-diameter, high-magnification scope can be a great help. Various manufacturers create standard rifle scopes that may allow people who are strongly nearsighted or people with a lack of visual acuity to shoot far above the level they could expect without the sighting aid.

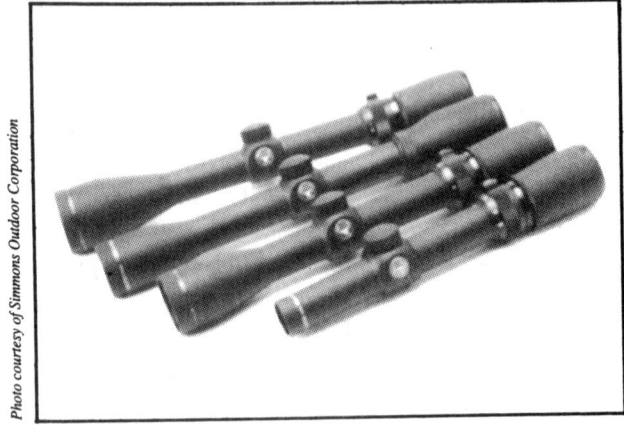

*Photo courtesy of Simmons Outdoor Corporation*

Since they won't be able to see holes in a paper target until they are retrieved, people with visual impairments will enjoy shooting targets that make a distinctive sound or disappear when hit. Using balloons for multiple bull's-eyes, metallic silhouettes for both pistols and rifles, and outdoor and indoor archery silhouettes prove exciting for all shooters.

### Aimpoint-Type Scopes on Rifles

An Aimpoint-type scope for pistols, rifles and shotguns projects a red dot onto the lens. In most cases there is no magnification, although 1x or 2x in power is an option on several models. These scopes typically use a longer eye relief allowing the scope to be mounted farther forward on the gun where it is easier for some shooters to see. The intensity and width of the dot is adjustable, and sunscreens can be placed on the front lens to make the dot show up better. While not the solution for everyone, they can be helpful to some.

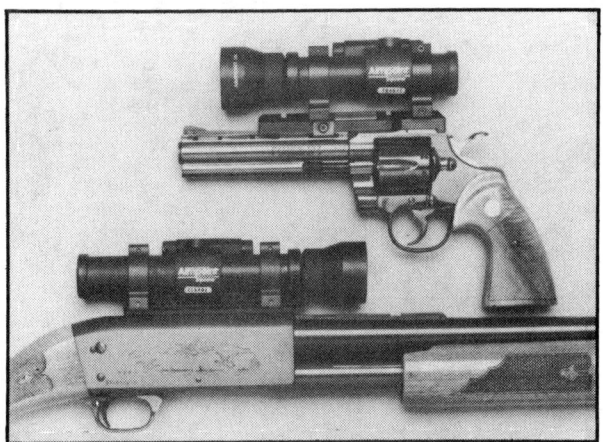

*Aimpoint-Type Scopes*

### Laser Scopes

Rather than making a dot appear inside a scope, a laser scope actually projects a dot onto the target itself. For people who are farsighted, this kind of sighting system can make a real difference in their shooting. The shooter only needs to be able to see the target and the red dot — anything else (including focus) is extra.

### Sightless Sight Systems

For shooters with visual disabilities, sightless sight systems, using sound waves, are available. A variation of this system is for students that also have a hearing disability. That disability is overcome with tremendous success by using a vibrating head-set.

### Tripod Gun Holder

The tripod gun holder, which is basically a modified camera tripod, lets students who have limited strength or control of their arms participate. By supporting the weight of the gun, the tripod gun holder gives the shooter the ability to aim and pivot to a small degree.

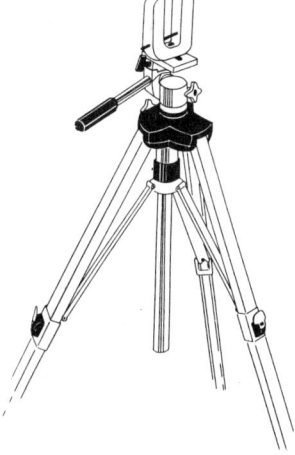

To make one, start with a strongly-built camera tripod. Bend a flat piece of steel (1/2" by 5/8" by 11") into a U-shaped holder for the fore-end or barrel of the gun. Weld or bolt the U to the top of the tripod and line it with a soft cloth padding. A large upside down U-bolt will also work as a barrel holder.

### Wheelchair Shooting Frames or Lapboards

Basically a wheelchair version of the above tripod gun holder, this shooting aid attaches to the chair frame. Support posts, ammunition holders, gun racks and squeeze device holders can be easily attached to the lapboard or shooting frame. There are many versions of shooting frames — some with tri-pod type supports and others which use the same attachments as for wheelchair armrests.

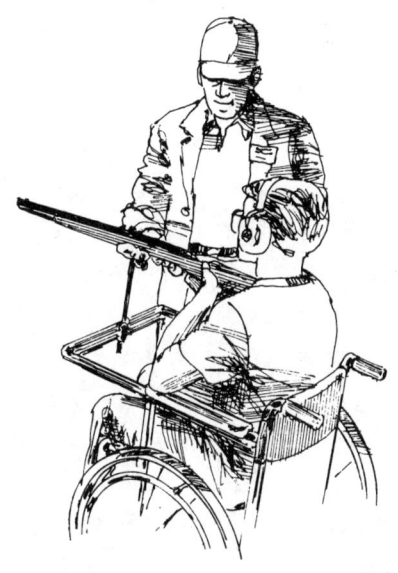

## Gun Caddy

A soup can or similar container attached to the legs of the wheelchair combined with a simple hook or loop can help wheelchair users transport their firearms. Mount the can near the floor and line it with soft material to protect the sights and prevent scratches. If the student prefers to have the muzzle up, use a can large enough to contain the stock.

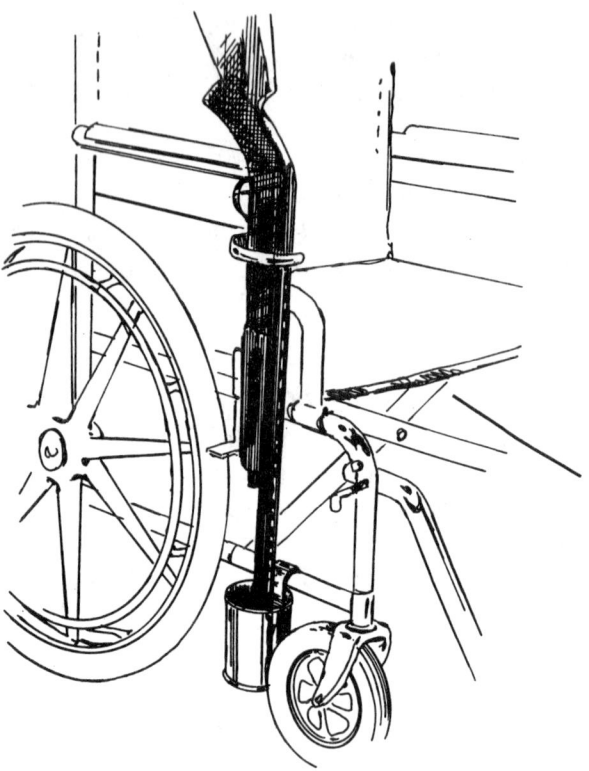

*Gun caddy made from a soup can*

## Squeeze Devices

Some students, for one reason or another, cannot operate a trigger in the regular manner. A wide variety of trigger aids are available or can be made to make operating the trigger easier. For example, a pencil inserted in front of the trigger may be used as a trigger squeeze device by someone lacking finger dexterity. A shoelace, tied to the trigger, can also serve as a trigger for someone without the use of their arms.

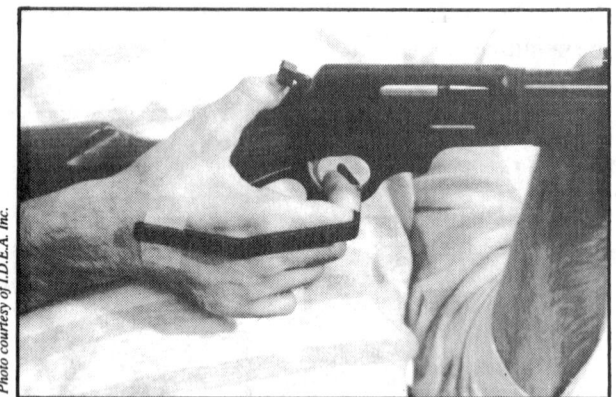

*Trigger squeeze can be assisted with a variety of devices, including this curved rod, which bends the index finger into a position where it can safely engage the trigger.*

Many shooters use a curved rod that can be strapped to their arm. The curved portion of the rod is placed on the trigger and the shooter then pulls the arm back while the hook pulls the trigger. There are electronic triggers which will offer increased adjustments as well as smoothness. Quadriplegics with little or no movement in their arms or hands have found ways to mount the firearm (attached directly to a helmet or to a shoulder harness) and then use a suck/blow tube in the mouth attached to an air switch and tubular solenoid that actually pulls the trigger.

## SR-77 Gunrest

The SR-77 is a combination shooting frame and shooting system which allows quadriplegics to shoot using a joystick and suck tube. A modified rifle rides in a special carriage attached to the armrests of a wheelchair. Automobile power-window motors controlled by a joystick aim the gun, and a solenoid, tripped by inhaling through a tube, fires it. The SR-77 is heavy and expensive, but allows quadriplegics to shoot.

There are dozens of adaptive triggers for archers. Many need no adapting while others may need to be modified for the shooter's particular needs. Some use a trigger method of releasing the string while others can release the string by simply lifting the finger off of a button. Self timing hydraulic releases as well as those held in the mouth are available depending on the shooter's needs.

## Sandbags

Sandbags may be used to help stabilize the rifle while students shoot. They are a must to steady a tripod and can also be used as wheel blocks for wheelchairs.

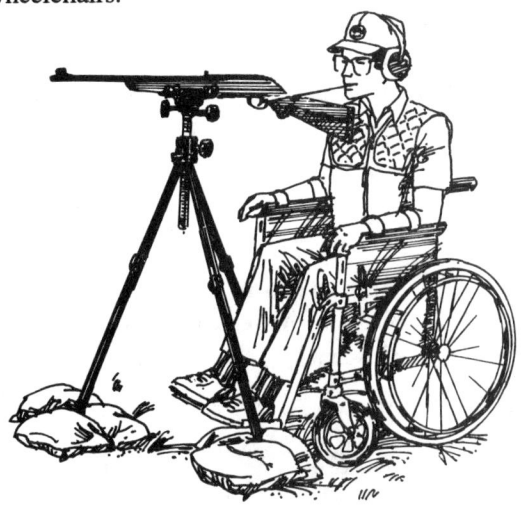

*Photo courtesy of SR-77 Enterprises, Inc.*

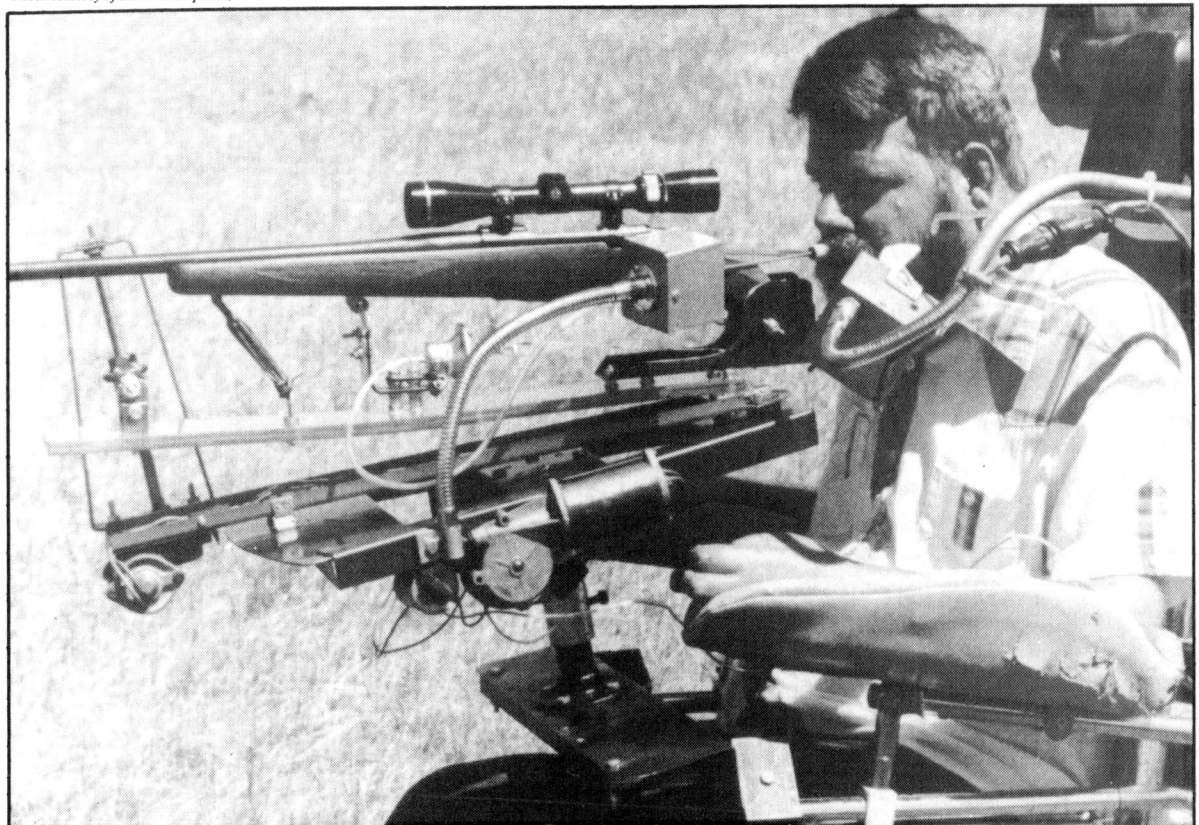

*The SR-77 gun rest enables quadraplegic shooters to zero in on their targets.*

## Cut-outs

Using construction paper cut-outs to show proper sight picture and sight alignment easily communicates the idea to many different groups of people. The cut-outs can be seen and felt and require very little translation, even if the student speaks a different language. (See full-size example of cut-outs at right.)

## Large Archery Targets

Starting with a large (easily seen) target allows the student immediate success — a vital component in the learning process.

## Blinders

There is a theory that leaving both eyes open leads to better shooting. Unfortunately, many people see two images when they try to leave both eyes open. To solve this, close one eye or use a blinder of some kind. Often, because of a disability, the shooter may not be able to use their dominate eye to aim and in these cases an eye patch or blinder is generally needed.

Translucent tape or masking tape placed over one lens of a pair of shooting glasses makes a very comfortable patch and can be used for a student that insists on shooting with his dominant hand rather than his dominant eye. Solutions for hunters include a pair of dark flip-up sunglasses with one lens removed, or a scope cover that flips out to block the view of the weak eye. Also, a blinder cut from a plastic milk jug attached to a target rifle's rear sight allows the student to leave both eyes open, and eliminates target confusion. A standard eye patch or gauze pad behind regular glasses works under certain conditions.

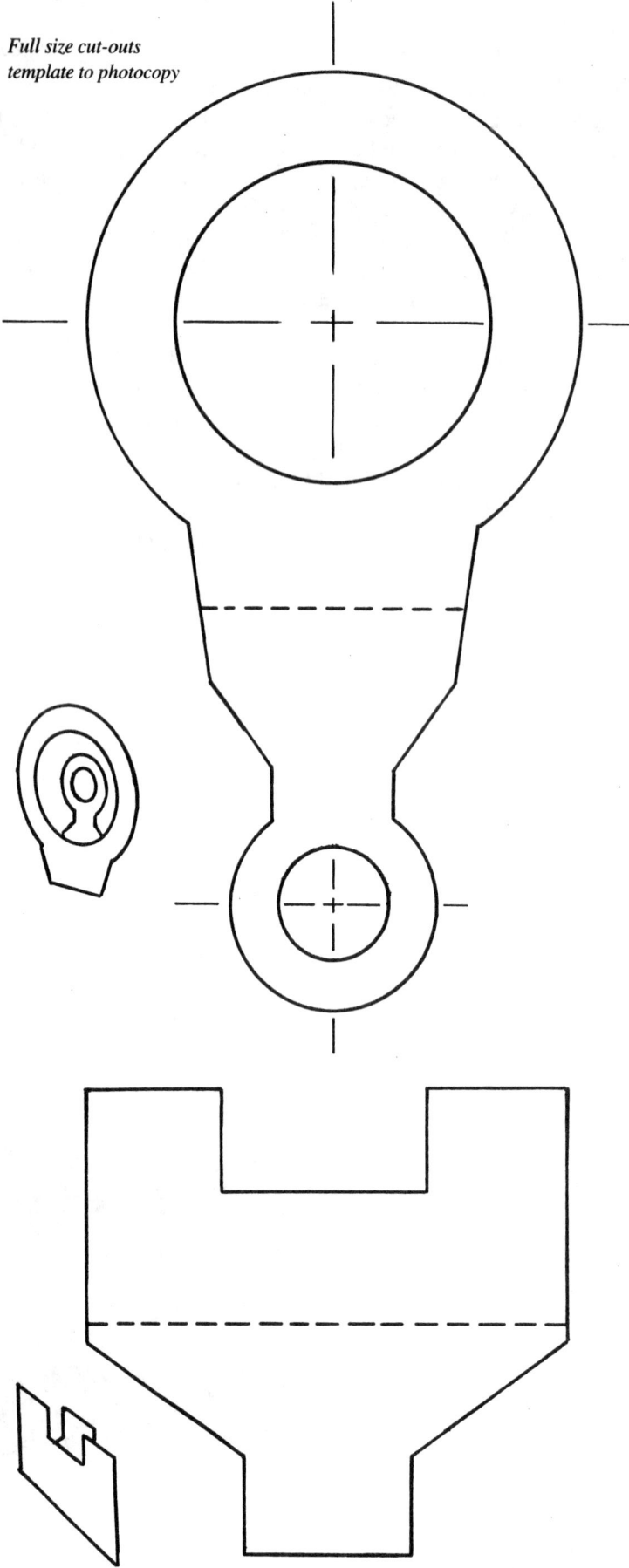

*Full size cut-outs template to photocopy*

# Riflery Lesson Plans

*(Each lesson plan in this book is complete and made to stand alone. You may find duplication in certain parts of each lesson.)*

**Materials needed:**
- Firearms
- Air rifles (preferably at least one $CO_2$ type)
  Lightweight .22 caliber target rifle (preferably at least one larger, precision rifle)
- .22 caliber Ammunition and Pellets
- Targets (standard smallbore rifle and pistol, pellet, large bore, silhouette, scope sight-in and assorted novelty targets)
- Balloons
- Clothespins
- Sandbags
- Hearing protection
- Eye protection
- Visual aids (cut-outs)
- Repair tools
- Sunscreen (if appropriate)
- Insect repellent (if appropriate)
- Shooting benches (mats if unavailable)
- Disposable plastic jug filled with water
- Water cooler
- Drinking cups
- Cleaning equipment
- Lapboard for wheelchairs
- Translucent tape and/or masking tape
- Rear sight mounted blinders
- Staple gun
- Staples
- Padding for bra straps
- Whistle or bull horn
- First aid kit
- Tissues

## Motivation and Introduction

For centuries hunting and shooting has been an important part of life for North Americans. Hunting helped sustain life as pioneers explored the frontier, and shooting is a recognized sport around the world, and a major part of the Olympic Games. Many organized youth groups recognize shooting as a sport which all students can readily participate in and actively promote.

**Instructor's notes:** For the student, competitive shooting matches provide an opportunity to both compete against one's self and to share in personal achievements, team spirit, and team pride in competition with others. Participating with a team can create feelings of unity between students and their peers and allow students to develop disciplined self-control.

As hunters and outdoor enthusiasts, the students' knowledge of shooting can enhance their enjoyment of the outdoors thanks to the many options shooting presents.

However, all students who participate in hunter education and shooting sports programs must learn to handle firearms safely and to practice safety in the field. When teaching any group, cover all aspects of safety thoroughly, including the careful handling of firearms in the home.

| Instructor Role/Activity and Objectives | Student Role/Activity |
|---|---|
| 1. Define and explain firearms. | 1. Students realize that a firearm is a tool. |
| 2. Identify the major parts of the rifle and their functions. | 2. Students examine actual firearms. They ask and answer questions. |
| 3. Rifle handling and safety:<br>   a. Determine dominant eye.<br>   b. Determine proper sight picture. | 3. Students test each other for dominant eye and with the cutout sight, demonstrate understanding. |
| 4. Name the three rules of shooting safety. | 4. Students share with other students the application of the three safety rules. |
| 5. Explain marksmanship, which combines all of the above skills. | 5. Students demonstrate skills learned up to this point. |
| 6. Demonstrate the steps for cleaning and storing a firearm. | 6. Students copy the cleaning steps and demonstrate their understanding of them. |
| 7. Explain the importance of eye and ear protection. | 7. Students try on different eye and hearing protection devices. |

**Conclusion:**
At the end of this lesson each student should:
1. Have reviewed the basics of shooting.
2. Have fired several shots.
3. Have helped to clean a rifle.
4. Leave with a good feeling about the class.

  A. Review:
    1. Safety
    2. Shooting fundamentals
  B. Shooting:
    1. Ask the students what they would like to do.
    2. Each student may shoot reactive targets, work on qualification awards, or try different positions.
  C. Cleaning:
    1. Divide the students into pairs.
    2. Assign each pair a rifle and have them clean it as they did in the last lesson.
  D. Farewell.
  E. Evaluation of the program by the staff.

## Sample Outline

A sample outline for a rifle shooting skills program that includes students with disabilities appears below. Modify the outline to fit particular needs.

**I. Introduction and safety.**
At the end of this lesson each student should:
1. Understand safe firearm handling.
2. Begin learning firearms vocabulary.
3. Be able to identify different rifle parts and action types.

  **A. Introduction of staff and students.**
  **B. Firearms safety.**
    1. Introduce the firearm safety rules:
      a. Treat every firearm like a loaded firearm.
      b. Always control the muzzle of your firearm.
      c. Be sure of your target and what is beyond.
      d. Know the range commands.
    2. Explain muzzle control.
      a. The muzzle is the front portion of a rifle barrel where the projectile bullet exits.
      b. Control is never pointing the rifle at anything you don't want to shoot.

**Ask:** Why is it important to point the muzzle in a safe direction?

  **C. Introduce equipment.**
    1. Identify the three major parts of a firearm.
      a. Stock.
      b. Action.
      c. Barrel.
    2. Have students identify each.

*Parts of a Bolt Action Rifle*

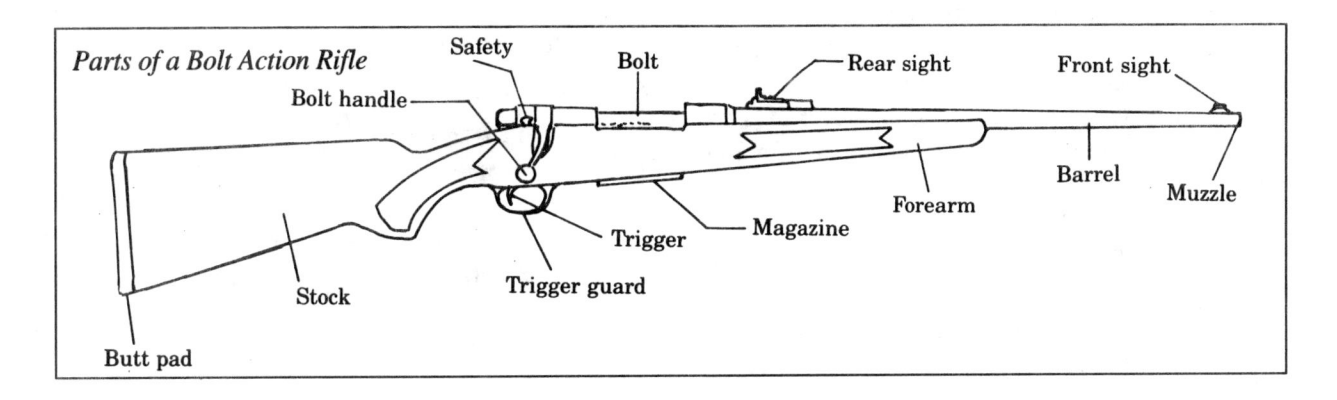

**Instructor's Note:** Allow students to touch or examine each part of the firearm.

**Student activity:** Have a simple bolt-action .22 taken apart into three pieces (bolt, stock, and barreled action) and let the students put it back together (or describe the procedure).

   3. Discuss the safety on the firearm and any adaptive equipment to be used in the class.

      a. Safeties are only mechanical devices, and can fail.

      b. Safeties can never substitute for safe gun handling.

      c. Demonstrate the use of the safety and point out that there are many kinds of safeties and that they all work differently.

      d. If possible, show several firearms with safeties and explain the differences.

      e. For students with sight impairments, show them how the safeties feel, rather than look, in the different positions (this applies to all activities with students with sight impairments).

**Ask:** When should the safety be off?
*Answer:* Just before shooting.
**Ask:** Where should the muzzle be pointed?
*Answer:* In a safe direction, usually downrange.

   4. Treat every gun as if it were loaded, and explain why.

      a. Close the action on the firearm, show it to the students, and ask if they can tell whether the firearm is loaded.

      b. If they say "Yes," ask how they can tell.

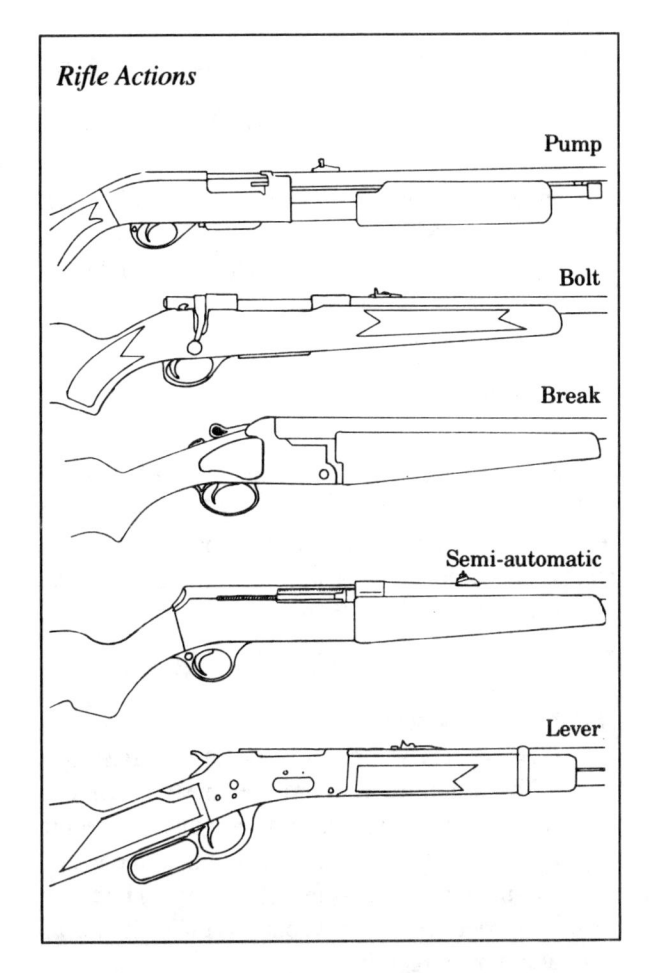

*Rifle Actions*

      c. If they say "By looking down the barrel," ask "Where should the barrel be pointed?"

      d. Convince students they should point the muzzle in a safe direction, then open the action to check if it is loaded.

*Rifle/Airgun Theory & Assistive Devices* 29

**Ask:** Why do we point it in a safe direction?
*Answer:* "Because we don't know whether or not it is loaded." Or "Because it could go off."
Repeat this exercise at every session. Never pass up the opportunity to stress muzzle control and firearm safety.

    5. Action types.

    Have examples of each major type of action open and displayed, preferably with labels on them identifying each by type.

        a. Explain how each style of action works.
- How to load.
- How to unload.
- How to make safe — locking the action open and checking for ammunition.

        b. Point out the hazardous areas of the action.
- Opening and closing of the break action could result in pinched fingers.
- Demonstrate how the carriage slams back and forth on the autoloader and pump.

    6. Ammunition
        a. Rifles shoot a single projectile.
        b. Demonstrate bullet impact.

**Instructor's note:** This demonstration will give the students a quick and positive idea of the difference between how a rifle shoots and how a shotgun shoots. This will be demonstrated several times in the following sections.

- Flashlight demonstration.
    - In the classroom situation, use a flashlight with an adjustable beam; demonstrate the difference between rifles and shotguns by shining a focused beam, then a wide beam, at the wall.
    - Explain how the focused beam (rifle) lights up the target very brightly, but it is difficult to keep a moving target lit.
    - Explain that while the wide beam lights up the target less brightly, it makes it easier to keep the target lit (refer to page 47).

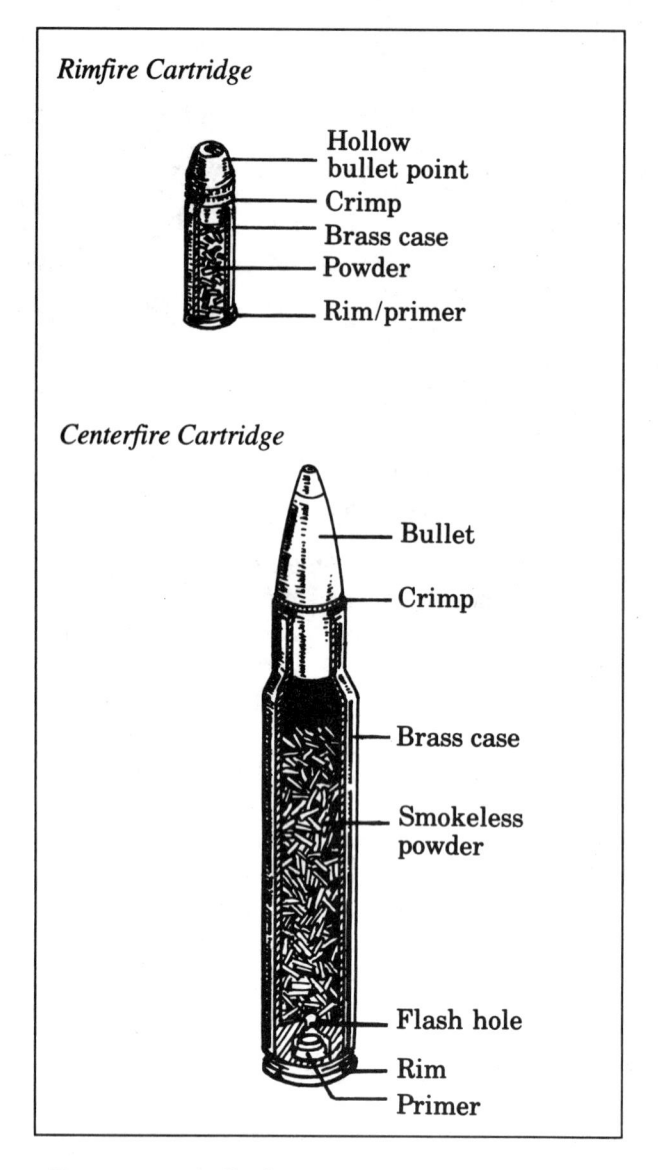

*Rimfire Cartridge*
- Hollow bullet point
- Crimp
- Brass case
- Powder
- Rim/primer

*Centerfire Cartridge*
- Bullet
- Crimp
- Brass case
- Smokeless powder
- Flash hole
- Rim
- Primer

- Demonstrate bullet impact on the range.
    - Place a plastic milk jug filled with water downrange.
    - Explain that the jug could represent a target.
    - Shoot the jug.
    - Open the action and lay the gun aside.
    - Ask the students what happened.
    - Emphasize the importance of muzzle control.
    - Repeat why they should make sure of their target before they shoot.

## II. Learning how to shoot.

At the end of this lesson each student should:

1. Know what eye they will shoot with. This may or may not be their dominant eye, depending on their specific situation.
2. Understand sight alignment vs. sight picture.
3. Understand the range commands.

### A. Safety review.

**Ask:** Where should the muzzle be pointed? Do safeties always work? How can you tell when the gun is loaded?

### B. Determine master eye, or the eye the shooter will be using.

(Shooters prefer, if possible, to shoot with their dominant eye. But, if because of a disability that makes it impossible, adjustments and adaptive devices can be used. The following section is for those shooters who will be shooting with their dominant eye.) The side of the body a given shooter shoots with is determined by their master eye, not by if they are right- or left-handed. Some students will be cross-dominant: right-handed but left-eyed. Teach them to shoot according to their eyes, not their hand, if at all possible. To determine dominant eye, use one of two techniques:

1. Paper technique.
   a. Hold a piece of paper with a ½" diameter hole cut in the middle at arm's length.
   b. Look through the hole in the paper at an object far away.
   c. Slowly pull the paper back to your face while looking through the hole.
   d. As the hole reaches your face, the hole will surround the dominant eye.
2. Two-hands technique.
   a. Face an object 10 feet away.
   b. Extend your arms out in front of you.
   c. Form a small triangle by overlapping your hands.
   d. Look through the triangle with both eyes.
   e. Focus on an object.
   f. Bring your hands toward your eyes, keeping the object in focus at all times.
   g. To keep the object in sight, the triangle will move toward the dominant eye.

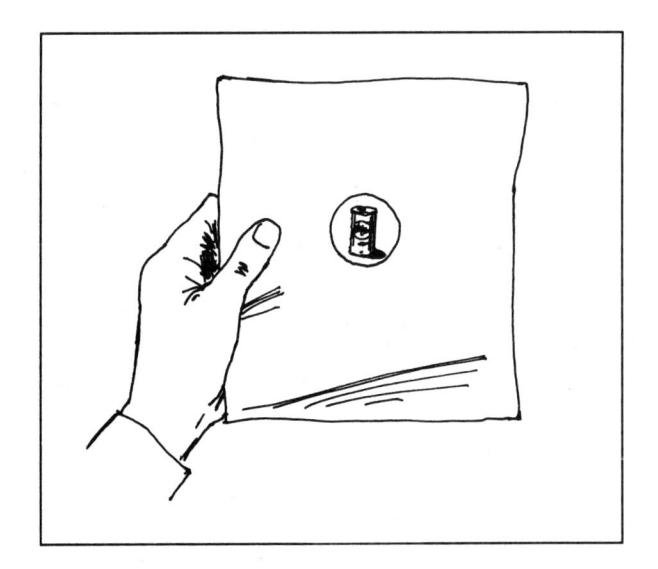

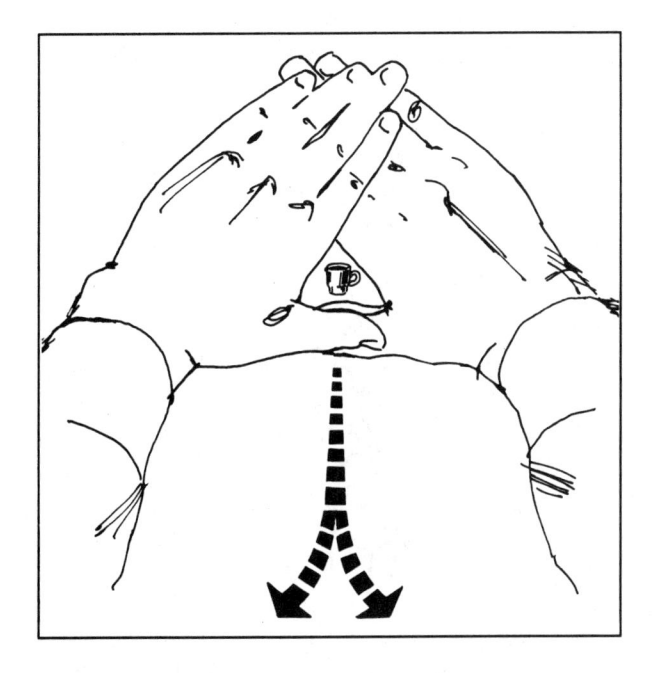

### C. Alignment and sight picture.

1. Closing or winking one eye.
   a. Leaving both eyes open leads to better shooting.
   b. Some people see two targets when they leave both eyes open.
   c. To solve the problem, either wink or use a blinder of some sort.

2. Sight alignment and sight picture.

   a. Explain "sight alignment" (the proper alignment of the front and rear sights relative to the eye) and "sight picture" (sight alignment relative to the target).

   b. Show students the front and rear sights.

3. Show students cut-outs of the front and rear sights.

   a. Hold them against the rifle to show which is which.

   b. Lay the rifle aside and have the students identify which cut-out is which.

4. Using the cut-outs, demonstrate proper sight alignment.

   a. Quiz students by placing the front sight too high or too low relative to the rear sight.

   b. Explain, using other cut-outs, the different kinds of sights.

5. Demonstrate how the sights should be aligned relative to the target (sight picture) using the cut-outs.

   a. Stress the importance of sight alignment.

   b. Repeat this exercise daily until the students demonstrate they understand sight alignment and sight picture.

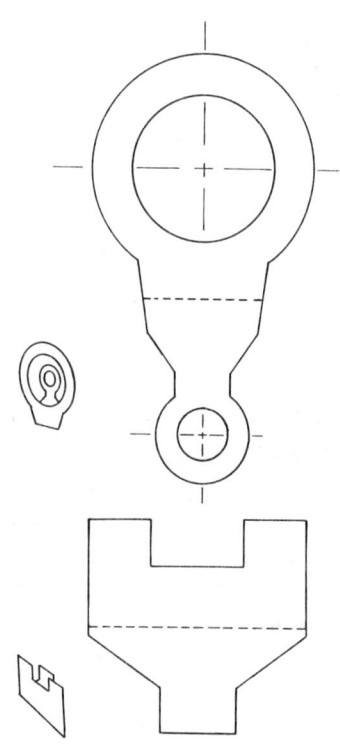

*See page 25 for full size cut-outs template*

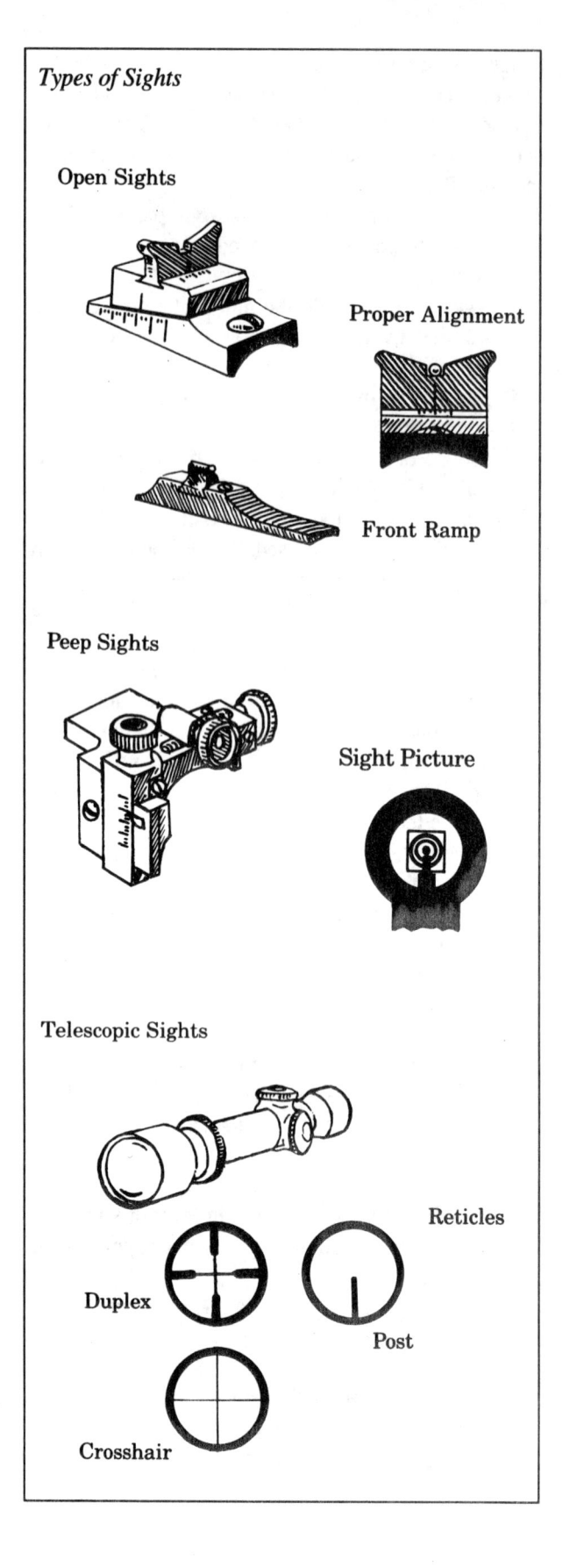

*Types of Sights*

Open Sights

Proper Alignment

Front Ramp

Peep Sights

Sight Picture

Telescopic Sights

Reticles

Duplex

Post

Crosshair

32  Rifle/Airgun Theory & Assistive Devices

**Student activity:** Have the students make their own cut-outs and practice with them. Make marks on the back where cutouts overlap to show how precisely the sights can be aligned.

**D. Shooting positions.**

The bench rest position is recommended because it is more stable and easier to adapt for use by people with physical disabilities. However, the positions used in these sessions will depend on both budget and the students' abilities.

   1. Explain the bench rest position.
   2. Demonstrate using a table and chair.

**E. Firing range practice.**

**WARNING:** If using dry firing as an exercise to teach students safety skills, trigger pull, and the workings of the action, take note. Dry firing some air rifles may seriously damage them. It is okay to dry fire pneumatic and low-velocity spring airguns. Many .22 caliber target rifles, shotguns, pistols and highpower rifles will also be damaged by dry firing without using "Snapcaps," a shell-like device which soaks up the impact of the firing pin. Check with the manufacturer of the particular firearm for their recommendations concerning dry firing. Otherwise, simulate the trigger pull with an uncocked firearm.

   1. Review how the action works. Include an explanation of the propellent system (cartridge, compressed air, $CO^2$).
   2. Pointing the barrel in a safe direction, simulate several shots explaining everything done.
   3. Have students repeat the demonstration.
   4. Range commands.
      a. Explain the range commands that particular range uses and emphasize generic range safety.
        • Demonstrate an audible "CEASE FIRE!" or equivalent visible signal and explain who can execute the command.
        • General rules: Never go forward of the firing line, no horseplay on the range, etc.
      b. Make sure all students understand proper range behavior and "CEASE FIRE!" or equivalent visible signal.

**Instructor's note:** If convenient, move to the firing line with assistants and position every shooter with a rifle, helping them mount the gun and find the sights. Otherwise, do the following in the classroom.

*Standard Shooting Positions*

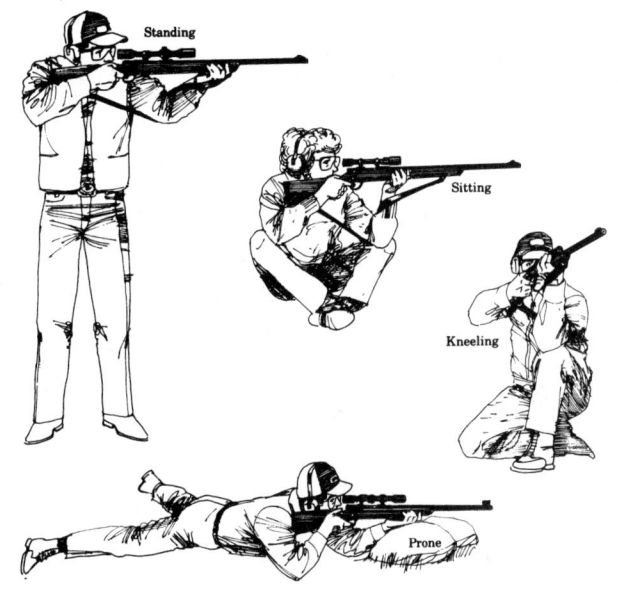

   5. Dry run.
      a. Choose which side of the classroom would be safest and announce that, for now, that direction is down range.
      b. Draw an imaginary line and allow small groups of students to simulate range practice step by step.
      c. If available, place tables and chairs to simulate shooting benches.
      d. Treat the whole affair with the seriousness due a real range.

**Instructor's note:** For the first few shots, be concerned about familiarization with the rifle and that everyone understands the range commands. Gradually introduce sight alignment, trigger squeeze, and sight picture as students become more comfortable. Toward the end of class, perhaps try a few "CEASE FIRE'S" to make sure everyone understands the signals, be they audio or visual.

### III. Firing the first shots.

At the end of this lesson, each student should:

1. Have demonstrated safe gun handling and safe behavior on the range.
2. Have fired their first shots.
3. Understand the importance of eye and ear protection.

#### A. Safety.

1. Review the three safety rules emphasizing muzzle control.

**Ask:** "Is this gun loaded?" "How do you know?" "Where should I point it?"

2. Using cut-outs, have the students identify front and rear sights, proper sight alignment, sight picture, etc.
3. Review the range commands and ask questions to make sure everyone — including assistants — understands.

#### B. Eye and hearing protection.

1. Expain the hows and whys of eye and hearing protection.
2. Demonstrate how each type is worn.
3. Allow students to handle the different types.

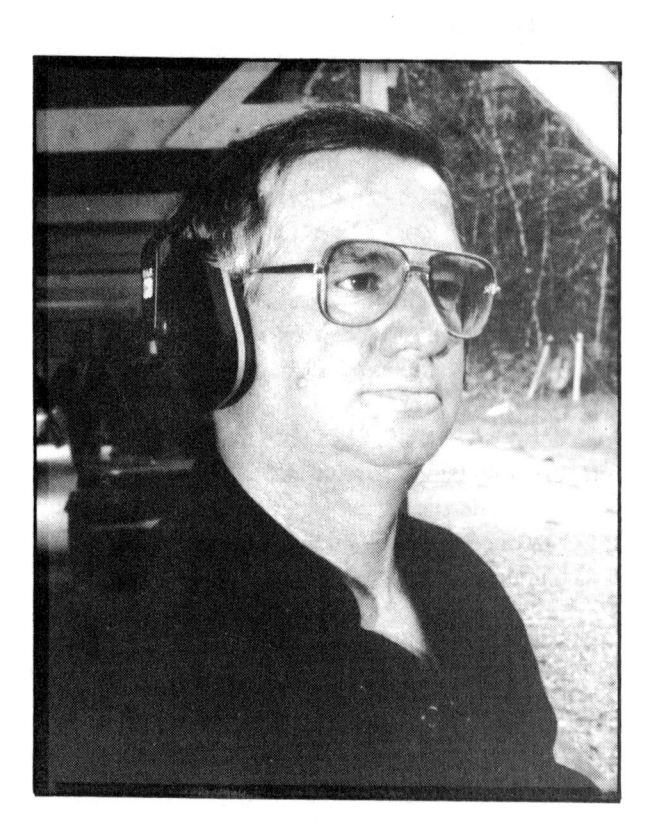

**Instructor's note:** Students with visual impairments and people with hearing impairments still need eye and hearing protection! In addition to being sensory organs, eyes and ears are soft and easily damaged. Protect their senses - have them wear eye and hearing protection.

#### C. Shooting review.

1. Gather students around one firing point where there is placed a rifle and ammunition.
2. Briefly review the fundamentals of firing a shot.
3. Go through the motions of firing a shot, exaggerating each action, including follow-through.
4. Repeat the above exercises with a live round.

#### D. Live fire.

1. Place the students on the line with an assistant. (Mother, father, brother, sister, grandparent or whoever accompanied them to class would make a good assistant. They not only give a hand in class, but they can be trained to accompany the student once they have graduated from the course. Quick students also make good assistants, and often they are flattered if asked for help.)
2. Try to have one student per assistant, particularly at this phase.
3. With the assistant looking on, allow each student to load one cartridge, and mount the gun to their shoulder, or other safe position.
   a. Make sure no one has their finger in the trigger guard.
   b. Make sure the students have the safety on.
4. Check if each student is lined up with their target. If necessary, stand behind students to help them find the target.
5. Talk the class through the shot. Emphasize sight alignment, trigger control, and sight picture.
6. After the shot, have the students make their rifles safe.
7. Check that the line is clear and show each student where their shot went.
8. Have each student fire at least twice more to get a group.
9. Rotate so all students get to shoot.

**Instructor's notes:** Give positive reinforcement for everything the students do right, even if they miss. After doing this exercise two or three times, allow assistants to adjust the sights of those students who are grouping their shots well. Be aware that emphasizing precise sight adjustments can discourage students who are not shooting as precisely, by focusing their attention on other students' success.

### E. Review.
1. Review the procedures the students followed and praise the students for things they did correctly.
2. Encourage each student to take home their best target as a memento.
3. Introduce the "ball and dummy" technique.

**Instructor's note:** This technique should only be used for a student who has developed a trigger squeeze problem — do not use for all students.

4. At the end of this lesson each student should:
   a. Have fired several shots.
   b. Have experienced the "ball and dummy" technique, if necessary (refer to instructor's note).
   c. Have participated in a shooting contest.

### F. Review.
1. Emphasize range safety procedures and muzzle control.
2. Take a break after 20 minutes or so.
3. Announce that after the break, there will be a group-sized contest.
4. Divide the class in half by counting off in twos.
5. Explain that each group of five shots will be scored according to the size of the group.
6. One shot on the paper scores 5 points, 5 shots on the paper scores six points, a grouping they can cover with a soda can scores seven points, etc.
7. Each student fires one five-shot group for score.
8. Score and tabulate the results.

## IV. Perfecting technique and shooting reactive targets.

At the end of this lesson each student should:
1. Have had assistance in perfecting their technique.
2. Have shot a reactive target.

### A. Safety review.
**Ask:** "Where should the barrel be pointed?" etc.

### B. Shooting.
1. Work on the finer points of technique emphasizing sight alignment and trigger control.
2. Introduce some games for those who are ready. Some examples are:
   a. Tape small objects to the target which will break when hit (lifesavers work well).
   b. Tie balloons to pieces of string, letting them blow in the wind.
   c. Arrange balloons in a grid allowing students to play tic-tac-toe with each other.
   d. Have a head-to-head group, or score contests similar to those done previously.

## V. Shooting and cleaning a rifle.

**Instructor's note:** If the class only uses air rifles, skip this lesson.

At the end of this lesson each student should:
1. Have fired several shots.
2. Have helped clean a rifle.
3. Understand the basics of cleaning a rifle.

**Instructor's note:** When cleaning, describe how things should feel and smell when they are clean. People with visual impairments won't be able to tell how a clean barrel "looks."

### A. Review
Ask: "Is this the safety?" "Where should I point the barrel?" etc.
### B. Shooting.
1. Refine technique on a case-by-case basis.
2. Stop shooting 20 minutes early.
### C. Cleaning.
1. Show the students how a dirty rifle looks, feels, and smells inside.
2. Contrast this to a clean one.
3. Assign rifles to pairs of students.
4. Slowly have them clean a rifle step-by-step.

**Instructor's note:** Remember, some cleaning agents are toxic and very irritating to skin and mucous membranes. Keep a close watch on everyone to be sure they stay safe.

## VI. Scoring and awards programs.
At the end of this lesson each student should:
1. Understand how to score a bull's-eye target.
2. Be aware of, or have begun shooting in, a rifle qualification program.
3. Have fired several shots.
### A. Review.
1. Safety, including range commands.
2. Parts of a firearm.
3. Sight picture using cut-outs.
### B. Targets.
1. Explain the different targets.
2. Explain scoring.
3. Explain how they work into any awards program used.

**Instructor's note:** The NRA offers a qualification program that has several awards. There is a cost, so be sure to inquire.

### C. Shooting.
1. Students shoot as before, but with minimum assistance.
2. Students score their targets with an instructor's help.
3. Reinforce each student positively.
4. Encourage each student to keep their best targets to show to friends and family.

## VII. Evaluate and clean-up.
A. Were the safety procedures followed?
B. Is the range clean?
C. Did everyone have fun?
D. Is all the equipment in?

## VIII. Evaluation of lessons.

# 7. Shotgun Theory & Assistive Devices

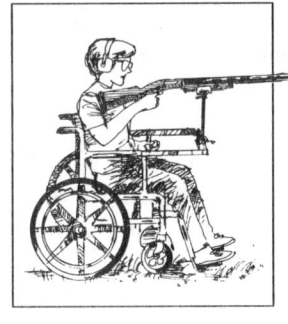

## Theory

Shotgun shooting games (trap, skeet, sporting clays, etc.) require a greater degree of physical mobility than rifle or pistol target shooting. But, even with this fact in mind, changes in the program and adaptive devices can go a long way toward overcoming any disabilities.

The recoil of a shotgun may appear to pose the biggest obstacle to learning shotgun skills, and using a smaller gauge (20, 16 or .410) shotgun would seem to solve the problem. In actuality, many times the opposite is true. A student wearing a good shooting vest with normal shoulder pads, shooting a semi-automatic 12-gauge with light loads, will have very little trouble.

## Shotguns

Although slightly more complicated than their pump or break-action counterparts, semi-automatic shotguns require less strength to operate on a shot-to-shot basis. Once the carriage of a semi-automatic has been locked to the rear, the only motions required to load and arm the firearm are loading shells into the magazine and pressing the carriage release button. Also, because they use their own energy to work the action, they tend to have less recoil.

Working a slide, cocking a hammer, and getting a stiff break-action shotgun to open have, in the past, been a deterrent to independent shooting by shotgunners with disabilities. Since semi-automatics cock and cycle themselves, they permit more shooters with little strength to shoot.

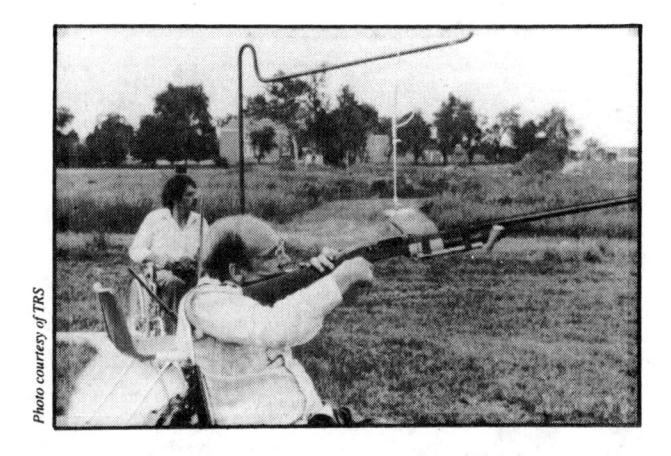

# Other Shotgun Options

A small .410 survival shotgun can help students with particularly short arms. A right-handed shooter with a short right arm can hold the shotgun against his shoulder with the right hand by gripping the frame. Trigger control and aim can be managed by the left arm. Adding a wheelchair with a lapboard and swivel, or an overhead suspension system, will give the shooter added stability.

For shooters who lack finger control and need to use their whole hand on the trigger area, the old Springfield Armory M6 Scout is perfect. The M6 Scout is an over/under .22 caliber rim-fire rifle/.410 shotgun. It is a break-top breechloader with a trigger bar rather than a conventional trigger. This design was originally intended for ease of shooting in cold weather while wearing gloves or mittens, which makes it ideal for shooters lacking acute finger control. Many of these guns are still available in used condition.

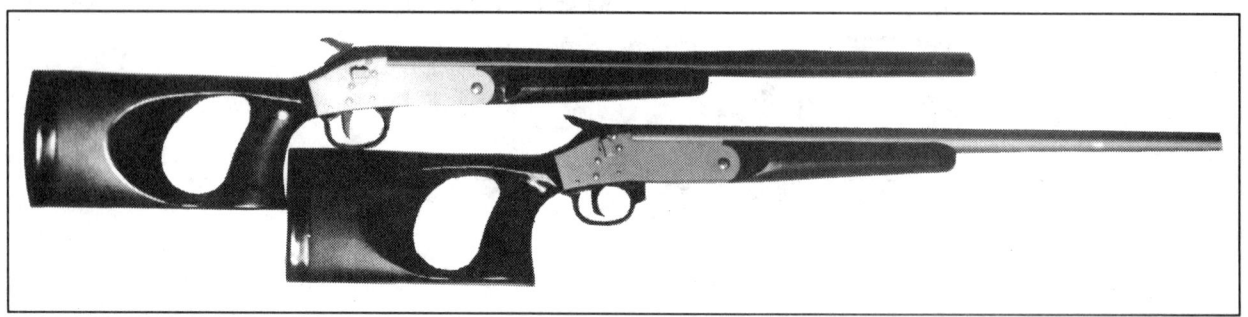

*Photo courtesy of Sporting Arms Mfg., Inc.*

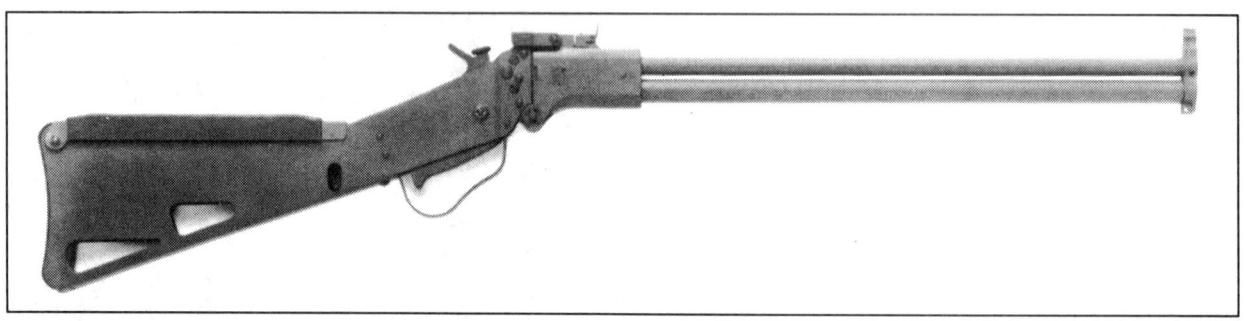

*Photo courtesy of Springfield Armory*

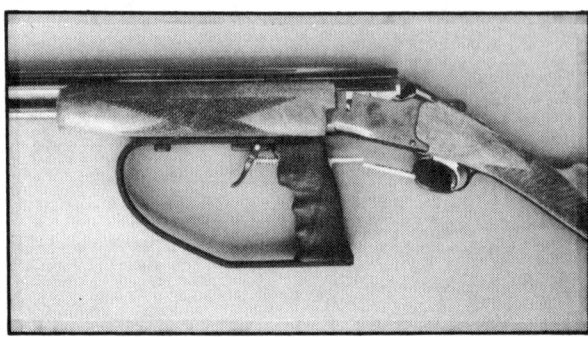

*Photo courtesy of TMS, Inc.*

Bullpups, or guns with the trigger mounted ahead of the action, work better for one-handed shooters than their barrel-heavy, conventional counterparts. With more of the gun's weight held close to the body, Bullpups are easier to control with one hand. Admittedly, there are few Bullpup shotguns on the market, but a standard break-action shotgun can be converted by mounting a pistol grip on the front end. The shotgun pictured here was converted by Therapeutic Recreation Systems, Inc. of Boulder, Colorado. For an explanation of how to do the conversion, contact them at the address listed in the Appendix.

Thompson/Center Arms sells a carbine stock conversion kit for their Contender line of pistols. Recently, Thompson/Center Arms began making .45 Colt/.410 shotgun barrels to fit the Contender which when combined with the carbine stock, yield an excellent all-around gun for someone with limited use of their arms.

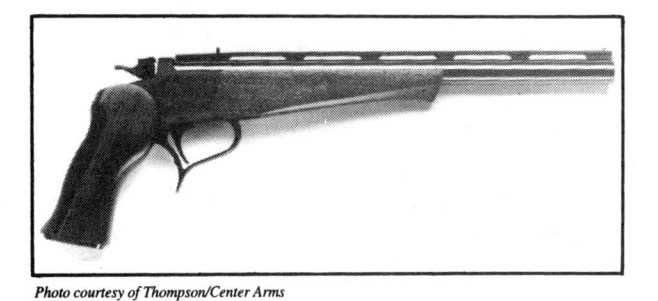

*Photo courtesy of Thompson/Center Arms*

## Assistive Devices

### Pistol Grip or Thumbhole Stocks

In some situations, pistol grips make it easier to hold rifles and shotguns in place. Thumbholes work well, but be careful that the thumb has plenty of clearance around the knuckles to prevent bruising from the recoil.

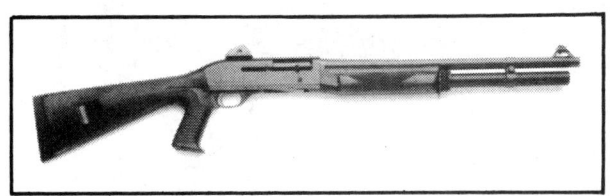

*Photo courtesy Heckler & Koch, Inc.*

### Trap Suspension Systems

An overhead suspension system or a modified camera tripod with swivel (see Rifle/Airgun Theory and Devices) will help students who might otherwise be unable to support the weight of the shotgun.

One trap aid is produced by Therapeutic Recreation Systems, Inc. They've developed a suspension system for all wheelchair users. A suspension rod fits into one of the vertical tubes housing the armrests on a wheelchair and supports an acrylic tube which surrounds the gun barrel. The tube swivels and can be raised or lowered onto the rod, which twists, offering a wide field of fire. An adjustable harness system holds the stock to the shoulder via a system of straps which attach to the shotgun's butt plate. A trigger extension system is available for those with impaired finger movement.

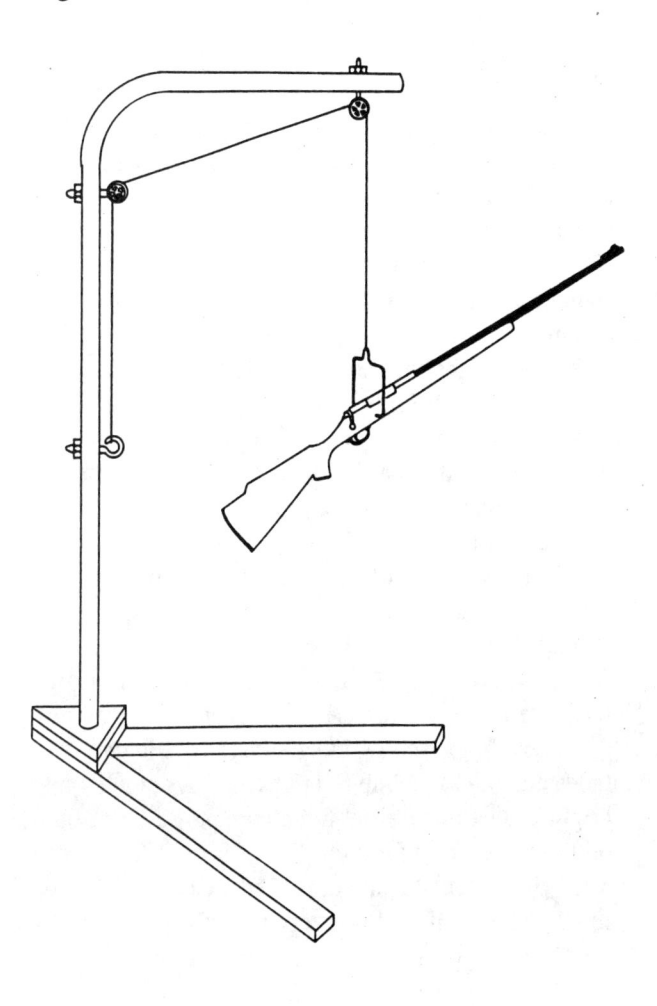

*Shotgun Theory & Assistive Devices* 39

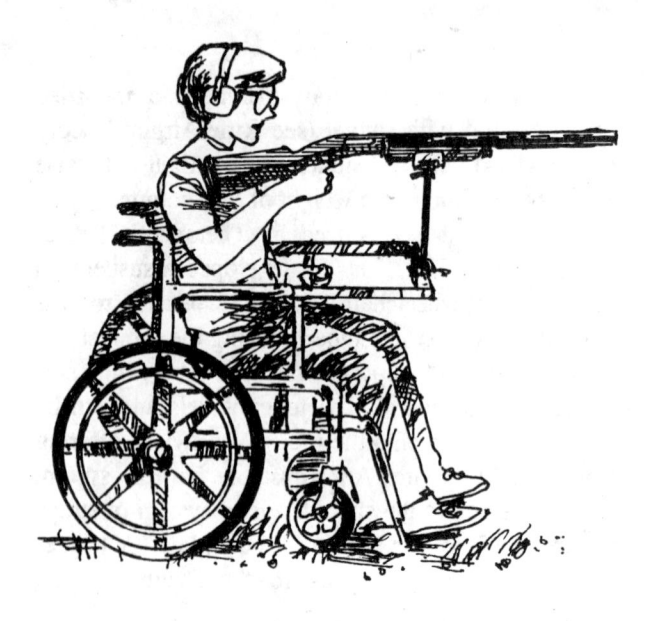

## Flashlights

Tape a small flashlight to a shotgun barrel or toy rifle and give it to a student to point at the wall. Shine a hand-held flashlight with a colored lens on the wall and have the student follow the beam with theirs. This works well for developing both stance and swing and can be done indoors easily, even outdoors at night.

If a flashlight with an adjustable beam is available, explaining the difference between a rifle and a shotgun becomes easy. A small dot puts a lot of light on the target, but it is hard to keep the dot on the target. A wide spread makes it easy to keep the target lit up, but it doesn't light the target very brightly.

Explaining the difference between chokes is just as easy using an adjustable beam flashlight. Full choke would be a small circle, improved cylinder would be much wider. If you walk farther from the wall, the brightness of the circle changes at different distances. Improved cylinder's circle gets bigger and fades out quickly while full choke's stays smaller and brighter. Just like a rifle, full choke puts a lot of light on the target from far away, but it is difficult to keep a moving target lit up. Improved cylinder lights up most of the wall, but not very brightly or from very far away (see page 47).

## Shooting Positions

There are many ways to help train students about shooting positions. For those students who will be standing at the shooting line, either provide a chalk mark for each toe, an outline of their foot or their own carpet square. Squares of carpet, with the person's foot position cut into them, can help show the person where they should place their feet when shooting in class or on their own. For shooters in wheelchairs, again chalk marks will work, or sandbags rolled up against the chair break with another one placed behind as a backup.

## SUSTAINED LEAD
1. *Point the shotgun ahead of the game, then swing.*
2. *Pull the trigger.*
3. *Fire.*
4. *Keep swinging after the shot.*

## SWING THROUGH LEAD
1. *Follow the flight path of the game until the firearm muzzle passes it.*
2. *Pull the trigger.*
3. *Continue the swing after the shot.*

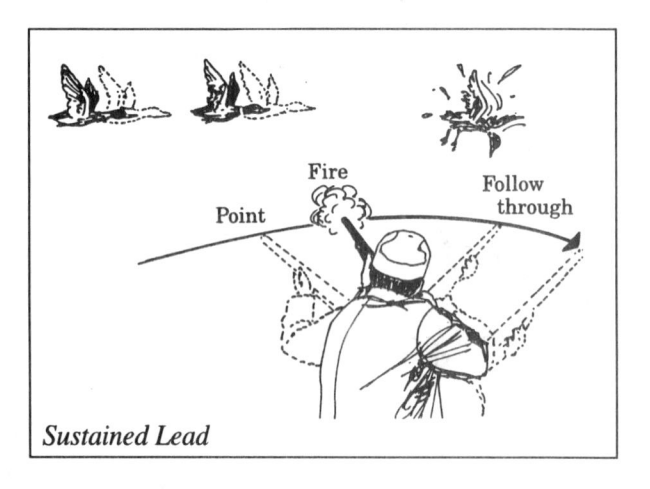

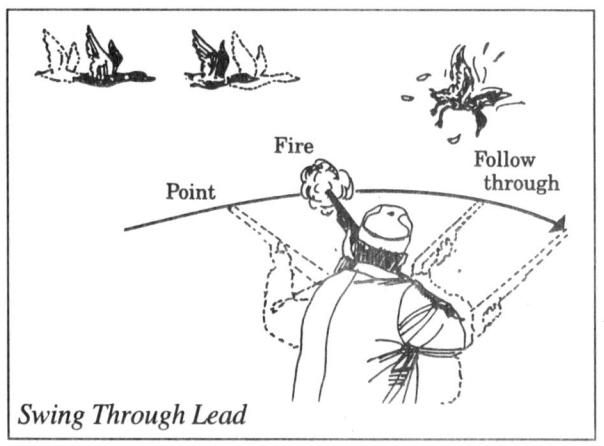

*Sustained Lead*

*Swing Through Lead*

40  *Shotgun Theory & Assistive Devices*

# Shotgun Lesson Plans

*(Each lesson plan in this book is complete and made to stand alone. You may find duplication in certain parts of each lesson.)*

**Materials needed:**
- Shotguns (one pump, one autoloader and one break-action of assorted gauges)
- Ammunition for all of the above
- Pattern targets and clay targets
- Balloons
- Clothespins
- Sandbags
- Hearing protection
- Eye protection
- Repair tools
- Sunscreen (if appropriate)
- Insect repellent (if appropriate)
- Disposable plastic jug filled with water
- Adjustable-beam flashlight and several small flashlights (optional)
- Water cooler
- Drinking cups
- Shotgun cleaning equipment
- Lapboard for wheelchairs
- Translucent tape and/or masking tape
- Staple gun and staples
- Padding for bra straps
- Whistle or bull horn
- First aid kit
- Hand thrower or portable trap
- Inexpensive frisbees (optional)
- Small football or tennis ball (optional)
- Ping-pong balls (optional)
- Water gun (preferably battery-powered) or garden hose
- Tissues.

---

## Motivation and Introduction

In early North America, blackpowder smoothbore firearms could shoot either a charge of shot (multiple pellets) or a single round ball. Later, rifling was added to the modern firearm barrel to increase the accuracy of the single projectile at long range. To this day, modern smoothbores shooting a charge of shot, continues to be popular for small game and waterfowl — as is the smoothbore, loaded with the modern version of the round ball or slug for big game.

**Instructor's note:** For the student, competitive shooting matches provide an opportunity to both compete against one's self and to share in personal achievements, team spirit and team pride. Participating with a team can create feelings of unity between students and their peers and allow students to develop disciplined self-control.

As hunters and outdoor enthusiasts, the students' knowledge of shooting can enhance their enjoyment of the outdoors thanks to the many options shooting presents.

However, all students who participate in hunter education and shooting sports programs must learn to handle firearms safely and to practice safety in the field. When teaching any group, cover all aspects of safety thoroughly, including the careful handling of firearms in the home.

| **Instructor Role/Activity and Objectives** | **Student Role/Activity** |
|---|---|
| 1. Define and explain firearms. | 1. Students realize that a shotgun is a tool. |
| 2. Identify the major parts of the shotgun and their functions. | 2. Students examine actual shotguns. They ask and answer questions. |
| 3. Shotgun handling and safety:<br>  a. Determine dominant eye.<br>  b. Determine proper sight picture. | 3. Students test each other for dominant eye and with the cutout sight, demonstrate understanding. |
| 4. Name the three rules of shooting safety. | 4. Students share with other students the application of the three rules of shooting safety. |
| 5. Explain marksmanship, which combines all of the above skills. | 5. Students demonstrate skills learned up to this point. |
| 6. Demonstrate the steps for cleaning and storing a shotgun. | 6. Students copy the cleaning steps and demonstrate their understanding of them. |
| 7. Explain the importance of eye and ear protection. | 7. Students try on different eye and hearing protection devices. |

**Conclusion:** At the end of this lesson each student should:
1. Have reviewed the basics of shooting.
2. Have fired several shots.
3. Have helped to clean a shotgun.
4. Leave with a good feeling about the class.

A. Review:
  1. Safety
  2. Shooting fundamentals
  3. Action types
  4. Other topics as per the instructor's discretion.
B. Repeat the shooting and cleaning portions of previous lessons.
C. Farewell.
D. Evaluation of the program by the staff.

## Sample Outline

A sample outline for a shotgun shooting skills program that includes students with disabilities appears below. Modify the outline to fit particular needs.

**I. Introduction and safety.**
At the end of this lesson each student should:
1. Understand safe firearm handling.
2. Begin learning shotgun vocabulary.
3. Be able to identify different shotgun parts and action types.
4. Understand the difference between a rifle and a shotgun.

  **A. Introduction of staff and students.**
  **B. Firearms safety.**
    1. Introduce the firearm safety rules:
      a. Treat every firearm like a loaded firearm.
      b. Always control the muzzle of your firearm.
      c. Be sure of your target and what is beyond.
      d. Know the range commands.

    2. Explain muzzle control.
      a. The muzzle is the front portion of the shotgun barrel where the shot exits.
      b. Control is never pointing the shotgun at anything you don't want to shoot.
**Ask:** Why is it important to point the muzzle in a safe direction?
  **C. Introduce equipment.**
    1. Identify the three major parts of a firearm.
      a. Stock.
      b. Action.
      c. Barrel.
    2. Have students identify each.

**Instructor's Note:** Allow students to touch or examine each part of the firearm.

**Student activity:** Have a pump action shotgun taken apart into three pieces (bolt, stock, and barreled action) and let the students put it back together (or describe the procedure).

    3. Discuss the safety on the firearm and any adaptive equipment to be used in the class.

        a. Safeties are only mechanical devices, and can fail.

        b. Safeties can never substitute for safe gun handling.

        c. Demonstrate the use of the safety and point out that there are many kinds of safeties and that they all work differently.

        d. If possible, show several firearms with safeties and explain the differences.

        e. For students with sight impairments, show them how the safeties feel, rather than look, in the different positions (this applies to all activities with students with sight impairments).

**Ask:** When should the safety be off?
*Answer:* Just before shooting.
**Ask:** Where should the muzzle be pointed?
*Answer:* In a safe direction, usually downrange.

    4. Treat every gun as if it were loaded, and explain why.

        a. Close the action on the firearm, show it to the students, and ask if they can tell whether the firearm is loaded.

        b If they say "Yes," ask how they can tell.

        c. If they say "By looking down the barrel," ask "Where should the barrel be pointed?"

        d. Convince students that the muzzle must be pointed in a safe direction, then open the action to check if it is loaded.

**Ask:** Why do we point it in a safe direction?
*Answer:* "Because we don't know whether or not it is loaded." Or "Because it could go off." Repeat this exercise at every session. Never pass up the opportunity to stress muzzle control and firearm safety.

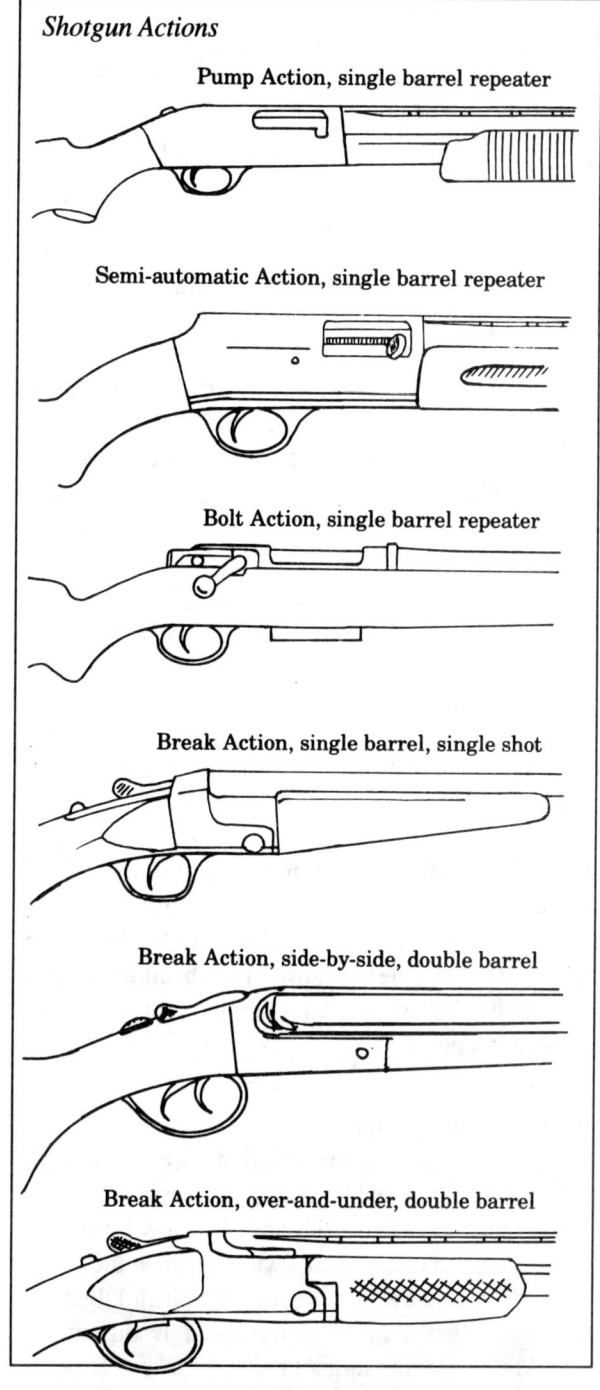

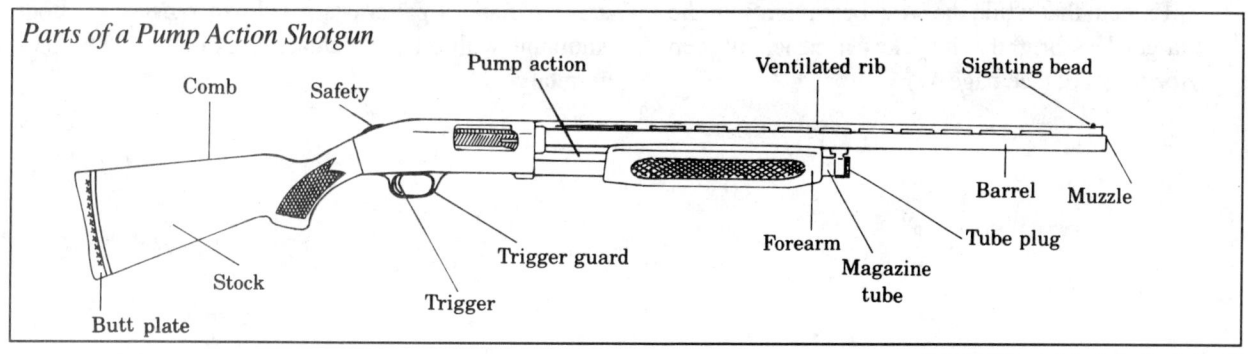

*Shotgun Actions*

Pump Action, single barrel repeater

Semi-automatic Action, single barrel repeater

Bolt Action, single barrel repeater

Break Action, single barrel, single shot

Break Action, side-by-side, double barrel

Break Action, over-and-under, double barrel

*Parts of a Pump Action Shotgun*

Comb, Safety, Pump action, Ventilated rib, Sighting bead, Barrel, Muzzle, Tube plug, Forearm, Magazine tube, Trigger, Trigger guard, Stock, Butt plate

Shotgun Theory & Assistive Devices

5. Action types.

Have examples of each major type of action open and displayed, preferably with labels on them identifying each by type.

   a. Explain how each style of action works.
- How to load.
- How to unload.
- How to make safe — locking the action open and checking for ammunition.

6. Sights.

   a. Point out the different styles of sights.

   b. If students ask why shotguns only have a front bead, or sometimes a center and a front, explain that the position of the shooter's head on the stock can serve as a rear sight.

7. Ammunition.

   a. Shotguns can fire solid slugs, single round balls or shot (many small balls at once).

   b. Have a shotgun shell pattern and impact demonstration.

*Shotgun Shell*

- Shot
- Plastic body
- Wad
- Brass head
- Powder
- Primer

**Instructor's notes:** This demonstration will give the students a quick and positive idea of the difference between what a rifle shoots and what a shotgun shoots. This will be demonstrated several times in the following sections. Demonstrate the difference between rifles and shotguns by throwing a whiffle ball (rifle bullet example), followed by a handful of ping-pong balls (shotgun shell example), at an object across the room.

• Flashlight demonstration.
- In the classroom situation, use a flashlight with an adjustable beam; demonstrate the difference between rifles and shotguns by shining a focused beam, then a wide beam, at the wall.
- Explain how the focused beam (rifle) lights up the target very brightly, but it is difficult to keep a moving target lit.
- Explain that while the wide beam lights up the target less brightly, it makes it easier to keep the target lit (see page 47).

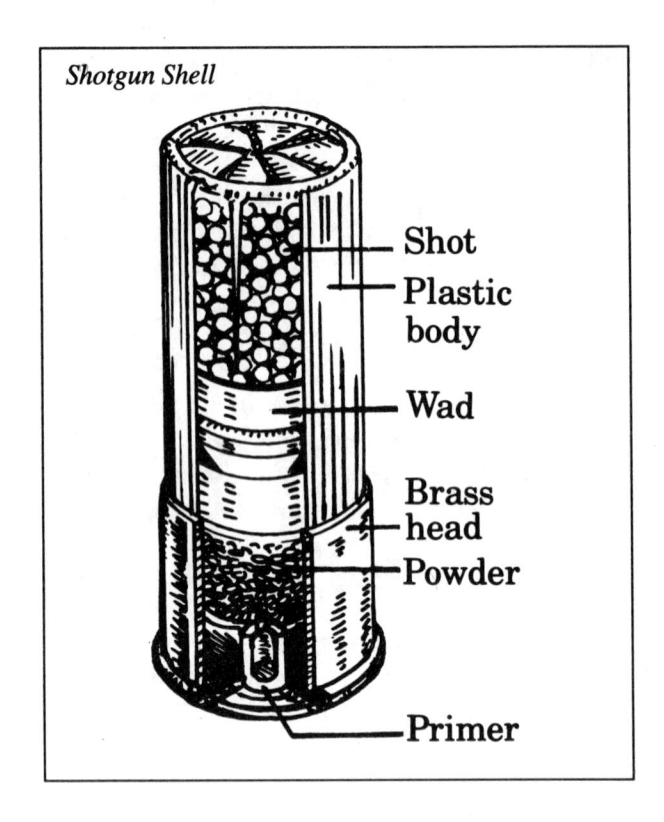

• Demonstrate bullet impact on the range.
- Place a plastic milk jug filled with water downrange.
- Shoot the jug.
- Open the action and lay the gun aside.
- Ask the students what happened.
- Emphasize the importance of muzzle control.
- Repeat why they should make sure of their target before they shoot.

• Next, hang a pattern target down range and shoot shotguns with different choke sizes into separate pattern targets.

44 *Shotgun Theory & Assistive Devices*

**II. Learning how to shoot.**
At the end of this lesson each student should:
1. Know what eye they will shoot with. This may or may not be their dominant eye, depending on their specific situation.
2. Have a workable stance and understand sighting down the barrel.
3. Understand "Pull," "CEASE FIRE" and other range commands.

**A. Safety review.**

**Ask:** Where should the muzzle be pointed? Do safeties always work? How can you tell when the gun is loaded?

**B. Determine dominant eye, or the eye the shooter will be using.**

(Shooters prefer, if possible, to shoot with their dominant eye. But, if because of a disability that makes it impossible, adjustments and adaptive devices can be used. The following section is for those shooters who will be shooting with their dominant eye.)

The side of the body a given shooter shoots with is determined by their dominant eye, not by if they are right- or left-handed. Some students will be cross-dominant: right-handed but left-eyed. Teach them to shoot according to their eyes, not their hand, if at all possible.

To determine dominant eye, use one of two techniques:

1. Paper technique.
   a. Hold a piece of paper with a ½" diameter hole cut in the middle at arm's length.
   b. Look through the hole in the paper at an object far away.
   c. Slowly pull the paper back to your face while looking through the hole.
   d. As the hole reaches your face, the hole will surround the dominant eye.

2. Two-hands technique.
   a. Face an object 10 feet away.
   b. Extend your arms out in front of you.
   c. Form a small triangle by overlapping your hands.
   d. Look through the triangle with both eyes.
   e. Focus on an object.
   f. Bring your hands toward your eyes, keeping the object in focus at all times.
   g. To keep the object in sight, the triangle will move toward the dominant eye.

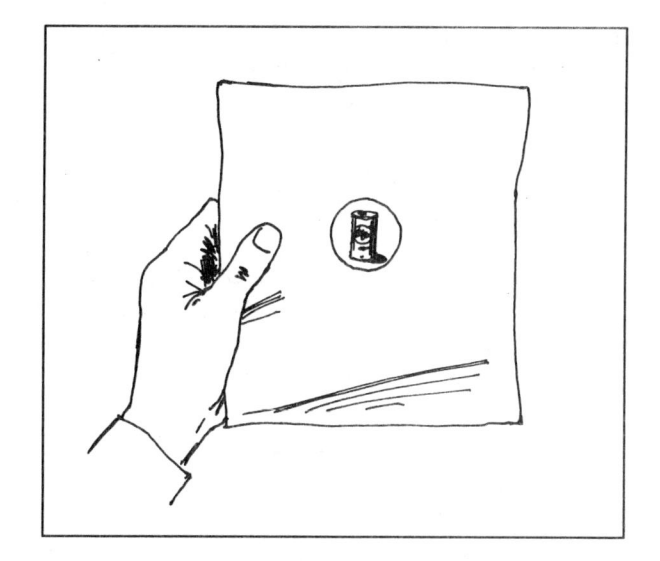

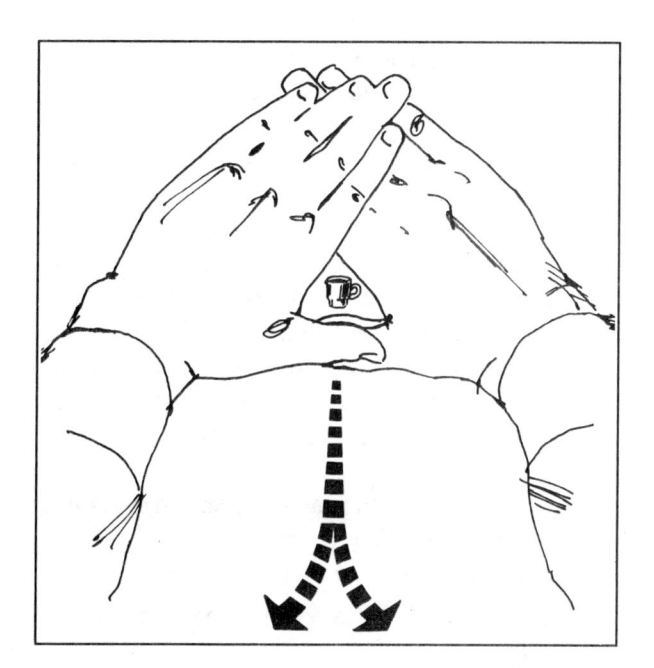

**C. Alignment and sight picture.**
1. Closing or winking one eye.
   a. Leaving both eyes open leads to better shooting.
   b. Some people see two targets when they leave both eyes open.
   c. To solve the problem, either wink or use a blinder of some sort.
2. Pointing the shotgun.
   a. Have an assistant demonstrate how to point a shotgun.
   b. As this is done, explain everything they are doing.

*Shotgun Theory & Assistive Devices* 45

**Instructor's note:** A training video can be very helpful here to show how national champions shoot in a fluid motion and follow through.

    3. Stance and pointing.
        a. Arrange the students on a line with their feet shoulder width apart.
        b. If the student will be using their right eye to aim, place the stock of the shotgun against the right shoulder, and move the **left** foot one-half step forward. (Shooting with the left eye, the procedure would be the opposite.)
        (Have wheelchair users treat the wheels of their chair as "feet" and place their opposite wheel forward by a few inches.)
        c. Take up a good shooting stance and tell the class to lean forward slightly, bending their front knee slightly. Keeping their shoulders square and upper body straight, they should bend slightly forward at the waist. (Demonstrate this pose while giving directions for those persons with hearing disabilities and manually position those persons with visual disabilities. Wheelchair position will be regulated by shooting style, either off hand or off a shooting aid.) When shotguns are used to check position, check shoulder and head position and make sure the student has a firm understanding of this before moving on.
        d. Have the students relax and then resume the proper shooting position.
        e. Walk back and forth in front of the group to readjust their positions each time you repeat the exercise.
        f. Check that the students swing their bodies as a unit, rather than swiveling at the shoulders or waist. Instructors should have the students point at their nose and follow it as they move across the room. Try the same by throwing an empty box across the room. Do it with up and down movements also. Wheelchair students using adaptive devices will see the extent of their swing. Students with visual disabilities will be able to start building timing from the time they yell pull until the target is in their swing line.

**Instructor's note:** This should be done in the classroom and at the range on a regular basis.

        g. Pick up an empty shell box and have the students point at that.
        h. Toss it lightly in the air.
  **D. Trap commands.**
    1. Explain "Pull."
    2. Demonstrate. Say "Pull" and toss the box across the room, pointing at it with the "aiming" hand.
    3. Explain the range commands used at that particular range.
    4. Emphasize the importance of "CEASE FIRE!"
  **E. Three parts of the shot.**
    1. Explain the action of the shot.
    2. "Swing" the shotgun to and through the target.
    3. Explain that to hit the target, they will have to be aiming slightly in front it when the shot goes off.
    4. Continue swinging after the shot to complete their follow through.

Outside, hang a ball from a rope and let it swing in a wide arc. Then have each of them use either a garden hose or a squirt gun to see how far in front of a moving target they must aim to make the shot.

**F. Flashlight exercise.**

1. If there are enough small flashlights, tape flashlights to two or three unloaded shotguns or toy shotguns of about the right size. Most anything will work. (If there are not enough, skip this exercise.)

2. Shine a flashlight with a colored lens on the wall and have students try to cover the spot on the wall with theirs.

3. Move the beam in long arcs, like the path of a clay target, while an assistant perfects the stance of the students.

4. Get everyone behind a mock firing line, and have the students dry fire under close supervision as they follow the beam.

5. Behave as much as possible as though the students really were shooting a clay bird — have the students say "Pull," make the target appear, and have the students swing to it.

**G. Review range procedures.**

1. (If the flashlight exercise has just been done, skip this exercise.) Walk the shell box back and forth for the students, as though it were flying in slow motion.

2. Have the students say "Pull" to start, and "Bang" when they could have shot the box.

3. Encourage them to say "Bang" two or three times, if able. (Non-speaking students can twitch their weak hand instead of saying "Bang" and stamp their foot for "Pull.")

**WARNING:** If using dry firing as an exercise to teach students safety skills, trigger pull, and the workings of the action, take note. Dry firing most air rifles will seriously damage them. Many .22 caliber target rifles, shotguns, pistols and highpower rifles will also be damaged by dry firing without using "Snapcaps," a shell-like device which soaks up the impact of the firing pin. Check with the manufacturer of the particular firearm for their recommendations concerning dry firing. Otherwise, simulate the trigger pull with an uncocked fire arm.

4. Get everyone behind a mock firing line, and have the students dry fire or simulate firing under close supervision at a spot on the wall created by a flashlight beam.

5. Behave as much as possible as though the students really were shooting a clay bird — have the students say "Pull," move the target slowly across the wall, and have the students swing to it and dry fire or simulate firing.

6. Emphasize follow-through.

7. If the swing is stopped, the shot will pass behind the target.

**H. Practice at the firing range.**

## III. Firing the first shots.

At the end of this lesson, each student should:

1. Have fired at least 1-2 shots.
2. Understand the concept of lead.
3. Have the remains of a target they shot as a memento.
4. Understand the importance of eye and hearing protection.

### A. Safety.

1. Review the three safety rules emphasizing muzzle control.
2. Explain the importance of keeping different gauges of shotshells separate.

   a. Demonstrate by dropping a dummy 20-gauge shell into a 12-gauge shotgun's chamber.

   b. Show how the 20-gauge shell will slide forward and become lodged in the barrel.

   c. Show how a dummy 12-gauge shell will fit in behind it with potentially disastrous results!

### B. Pointing exercise.

1. Move to the range.
2. Review proper stance.
3. Again, use the water gun or garden hose demonstration to reinforce stance and swing to the students.
4. The instructor should move back and forth while the student tries to get the instructor wet.
5. Keep reinforcing that they have to aim in front of the target (instructor) or the water will pass behind them.

### C. Eye and hearing protection.

1. Explain the hows and whys of eye and hearing protection.
2. Demonstrate how each type is worn.
3. Allow students to handle the different types.

**Instructor's note:** Students with visual impairments and people with hearing impairments still need eye and hearing protection! In addition to being sensory organs, eyes and ears are soft and easily damaged. Protect their senses — have them wear eye and hearing protection.

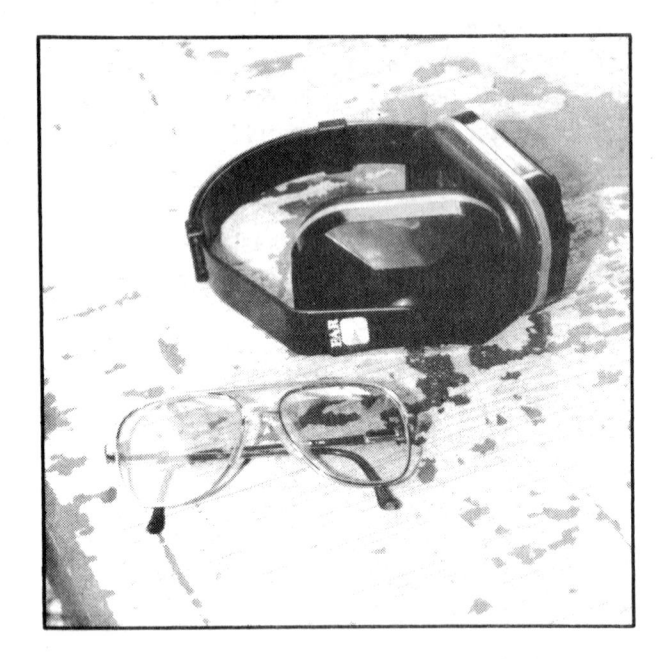

### D. Shouldering the shotgun.
1. As mentioned in the "Stance and position" lesson, shoulder position of the shotgun is critical.
2. The gun's recoil can cause pain or bruises if held wrong.
3. Arrange the students on the line at the range with unloaded shotguns.
4. Be sure every student has their gun well-seated in the pocket of their shoulder.
5. Check that their face touches the comb of the stock, preferably with slight pressure.

### E. Shooting the shotgun.

**Instructor's notes:** The noise and recoil of shooting a shotgun is often more of an obstacle than the idea of shooting a gun. Conquering this fear is often the main goal of the instructor. Whenever students are firing, the instructor should be the only person with ammunition. An eager student with an extra shell can easily lead to disaster.

1. Prepare to shoot a stationary target (plastic jug, milk carton). Students shooting from wheelchairs should lock their wheels, and sandbags can also be used as a wheelblock.
2. Suspend a milk carton or plastic jug from a target frame downrange.
3. Only load the shotgun with one round.
4. Carefully walk each student through shooting a stationary target.
5. Give the student the target to show what a shotgun can do.
6. If time allows, let students shoot at clay birds flying straight away, or at frisbees. Students shooting with an adaptive device and a limited swing need to know that they can hit the flying targets as well as anyone, within their swing limits. Students with visual disabilities will need to get the feel for proper height and swing timing. Work with them to squeeze the trigger at the same time as their swing. The timing is important and can be learned.

### F. Review.
1. Give lots of encouragement.
2. At this stage in the game, firing the shot is a big deal.
3. Reward students for their achievements.

## IV. Shooting moving targets.
At the end of this lesson each student should:
1. Have shot at a moving target.
2. Understand target thrower safety.

### A. Review safety and stance.
### B. Pointing exercise.
1. Graduate to having the students point at clay birds leaving the launcher.
2. Have a student call "Pull" (or stomp) to launch a bird for the group.
3. Have everyone point at the bird and say "Bang" two or three times (or nod their lead hand, as appropriate).

### C. Moving targets.
1. Throw and shoot frisbees instead of clay birds.
   a. For students in wheelchairs or using shooting devices, try to keep the frisbee flying straight away or at a slight angle.
   b. Waiting students should point at the targets as they fly away from the shooter.
   c. Encourage students to applaud and give encouragement.
2. After two or three frisbees, graduate to clay birds flying straight away.
   a. Brief students on target thrower safety.
   b. Show how it works.
   c. Stay clear of the throwing arm, and behind the trap.
3. Shoot at clay birds.
   a. Watch for signs of fear or pain.
   b. Always ask students whether they would like to shoot again.

**V. Emphasize "Swing," "Lead the Target" and "Follow Through."**

After this lesson each student should:
1. Have experienced the "ball and dummy" technique.
2. Understand choke.
   **A. Review safety rules.**
**Ask:** "Is this gun loaded? How do you know?"
   **B. Shooting.**
      1. Introduce the "ball and dummy" technique.

**Instructor's note:** This technique should only be used for a student who has developed at trigger squeeze problem and not used for all students.

   a. Instructors load the gun for the shooter with either a dummy or loaded round out of the shooter's sight.
   b. The student fires at a target, not knowing whether the gun is loaded or not.
   c. The instructor watches for flinching, lunging, or jerking.
      2. Repeat several times.

**Instructor's note:** This exercise can be fun for the other students to watch since even the best shooters in the class will lunge into the shot from time to time.

   **C. Review of technique, explanation of choke.**
      1. Discuss what the students have learned about shooting.
      2. Explain choke by shining a flashlight with an adjustable beam at the wall. For students with visual disabilities, choke cut-outs can be used.
      3. Explain and demonstrate how different amounts of "choke" focus the pellets into different sized areas by adjusting the flashlight's beam. Have samples of various shot pattern targets so students can see and feel the different sized choke patterns.
      4. If time allows, demonstrate the effect of choke on a shotgun's effective range by moving away from the wall without adjusting the flashlight.

   a. The dot created by a tight beam, or "choke," stays bright as it is moved away from the wall.
   b. The dot created by a wide beam quickly fades out.
   c. The brightness of the light indicates the number of pellets that hit the target.

**VI. Shooting and cleaning a shotgun.**

At the end of this lesson each student should:
1. Have fired several shots.
2. Have helped clean a shotgun.
   **A. Review.**
**Ask:** Where should I point the barrel?" etc.
   **B. Shooting.**
      1. Refine technique on a case by case basis.
      2. Stop shooting 20 minutes early.
   **C. Cleaning.**
      1. Show the students how a dirty shotgun looks, feels, and smells inside.
      2. Contrast this to a clean one.
      3. Assign shotguns to pairs of students.
      4. Slowly have them clean a shotgun step-by-step.

**Instructor's note:** Remember, some cleaning agents are toxic and could irritate the skin. Keep a close watch on everyone to be sure everyone stays safe.

When cleaning, describe how things should feel and smell when they are clean for people with visual impairments.

**VII. Evaluate and clean-up.**
   **A. Were the safety procedures followed?**
   **B. Is the range clean?**
   **C. Did everyone have fun?**
   **D. Is all the equipment in?**

**VIII. Evaluation of lessons.**

# 8. Archery Theory & Assistive Devices

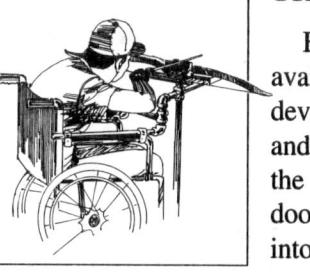

## Theory

By using lightweight compound bows and any of the multitude of adaptive devices available, most people can be taught to shoot a bow and arrow. The invention and development of the compound bow has literally brought archery to every man, women and child regardless of their age or physical abilities. In addition, the development and the full scale use of mechanical bowstring releasing devices has also opened many doors to new shooters, eliminating the need for strength or manual dexterity. Research into audible indicators has allowed accessability to the sport of archery for those persons with visual disabilities. It has advanced to the point of staging tournaments exclusively for those persons with visual impairments, including those people who are totally blind. With the full array of archery products on the market, many easily converted to use as an adaptive aid, the majority of people with varying abilities can now enjoy the sport of archery.

## Bows

The compound bow can look complicated to the new shooter, but in reality it is just a system of levers and pulleys. The compound bow could also be included in the next section on assistive devices. So, when speaking about the compound, it must be recognized that what makes this device so unique is that it is not made specifically for persons with disabilities. It is now the number one selling bow in the world for **all** forms of archery. The primary function that creates the difference between the traditional bow and the compound, occurs during the time when the archer is drawing the bow string back to their face (anchor point) and holding that position while aiming. As they pull the bow string of a traditional bow, measured as a 50 pound bow, the effort to pull the bow string increases until you reach the anchor point on the face. At that point the shooter is physically holding 50 pounds of pressure on the three fingers wrapped around the bow string. The compound bow differs to the extent that as the bow string is drawn back toward the face, 50 pounds of pressure is reached half way through the draw (at 12-14 inches into the draw). Continuing back to the anchor point on the face, the pressure decreases until the shooter is holding approximately 25 pounds of pressure with the three fingers wrapped around the bow string.

The advantage of shooting the compound for all shooters, including persons with disabilities, is there is no need to hold the heavier weight while aiming. There are the advantages of the higher weight in the shooting performance without the strain of holding the higher weight while aiming.

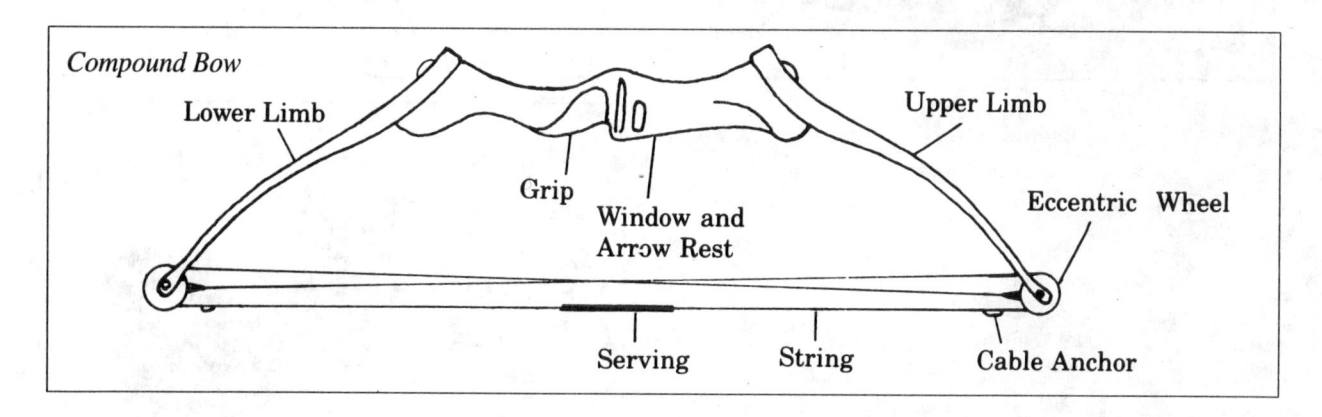

*Compound Bow*

Lower Limb — Upper Limb — Grip — Window and Arrow Rest — Eccentric Wheel — Serving — String — Cable Anchor

# Assistive Devices

## Assistive Devices for Hand and Wrist Disabilities

Amputees have dozens of mechanical bowstring release aids to use or adapt. The aids come with "T" shaped handles, wrist strap or a concho style. Their trigger mechanisms can be located on the top, bottom or straight out the back, with a variety of ways to attach them to the bowstring. Many of these devices can be mounted directly to a prostheses with little or no adapting.

## Elbow and Wrist Supports

These supports can run the full gamut from a regular archery wrist sling or duct tape, to a commercially manufactured support. A mechanical bowstring release aid can be used in conjunction with a support.

a. Wrist slings can be worn on the archer's bow hand or prostheses or attached to the bow. The sling's basic use for all archers is to keep the bow from falling out of their hand when shooting with a relaxed bow hand.

b. Commercial supports are manufactured for treatment of carpal tunnel syndrome and for use in spinal cord injuries. Products such as Thermo Plasti or duct tape can also do wonders in providing that extra support or confidence for the shooter.

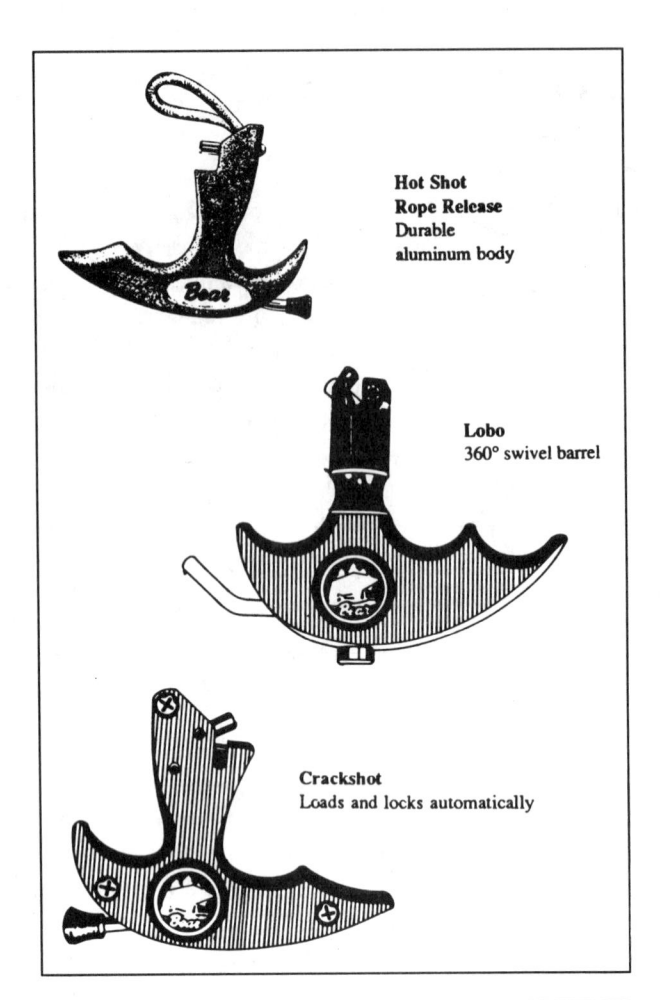

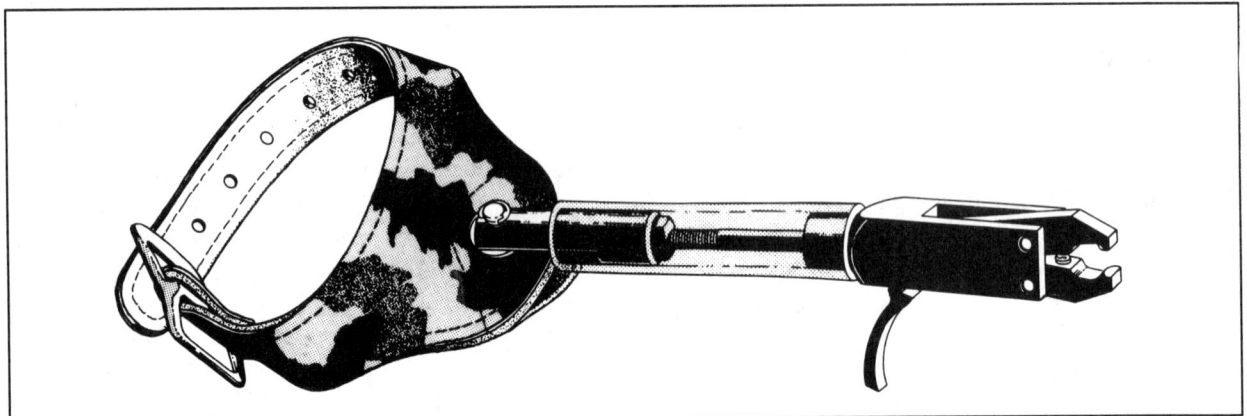

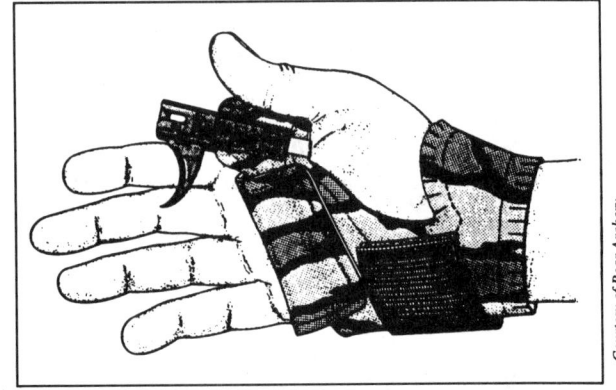

**Hot Shot Rope Release** Durable aluminum body

**Lobo** 360° swivel barrel

**Crackshot** Loads and locks automatically

*Courtesy of Bear Archery*

## Bow Supports

Although not accepted for competition in the United States Amputee Athletic Association or the National Wheelchair Athletic Association, the bow support can help many archers with disabilities. For those shooters lacking the strength to grasp or support the bow, stands designed to hold the bow upright in a shooting position have been developed. This particular adaptive device only holds the bow, but still permits the shooter to load, pull the string and release. It can be used for archers with little or no arm mobility using a "teeth tether" (a strap on the bowstring that the archers bites down on to pull and hold the bow at full draw while aiming. They release their grip on the "tether" and shoot the arrow by opening their mouth.) A teeth tether is also used by amputees with one arm.

Bow slings are another form of support for the archer of varying abilities. Straps attached to the bow can be slipped over the shooter's shoulder in a similar fashion to a backpack or a side bag. This permits the bow to stay with the archer at all times and also leaves both hands free for crutches or canes. This eliminates the need to lay the bow down after shooting or the fatigue of carrying it at all times.

**Note** There are devices which screw onto the bow that hold the string at full or partial draw. Check jurisdiction regulation concerning legality of use.

## Sight Systems

The "Sightless Sight System" enables archers with varying degrees of visual disabilities, up to total blindness, to shoot a bow and arrow very accurately. This is accomplished by using an electronic sound generating device.

All other archers can use standard sights with little or minor adaptations. A straight pin sight or a ring aperture works best in most cases.

Bowscopes and laser scopes might seem helpful, but in reality they can prove frustrating to all but the most experienced shooter. They tend to amplify the arm movement and are not legal in many states for hunting.

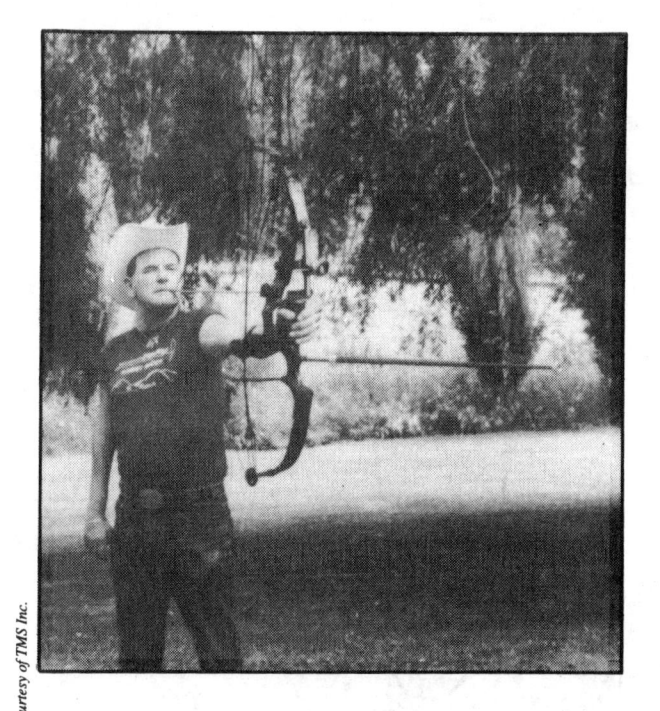

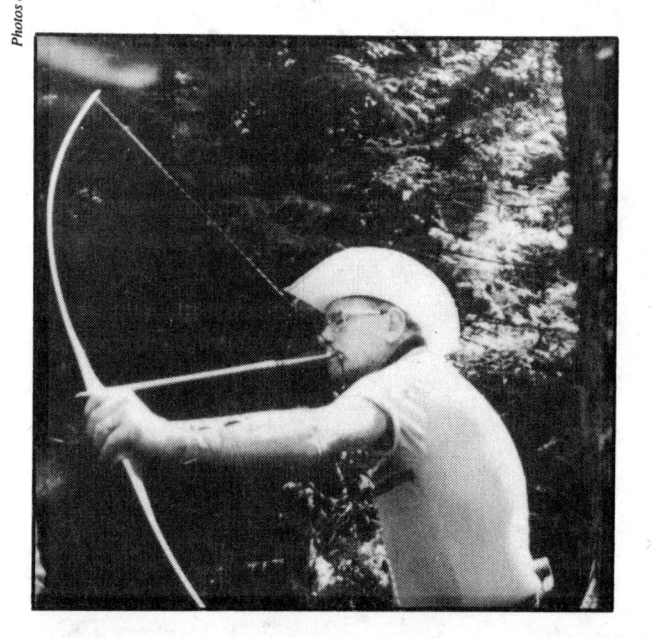

*Photos courtesy of TMS Inc.*

## Carpet Squares

For a student who needs foot or body positioning help while practicing away from the class, a carpet square with properly aligned cut-out footprints can help maintain foot position. For the average shooter, strips of masking tape on the floor is enough to reinforce proper foot position during the class.

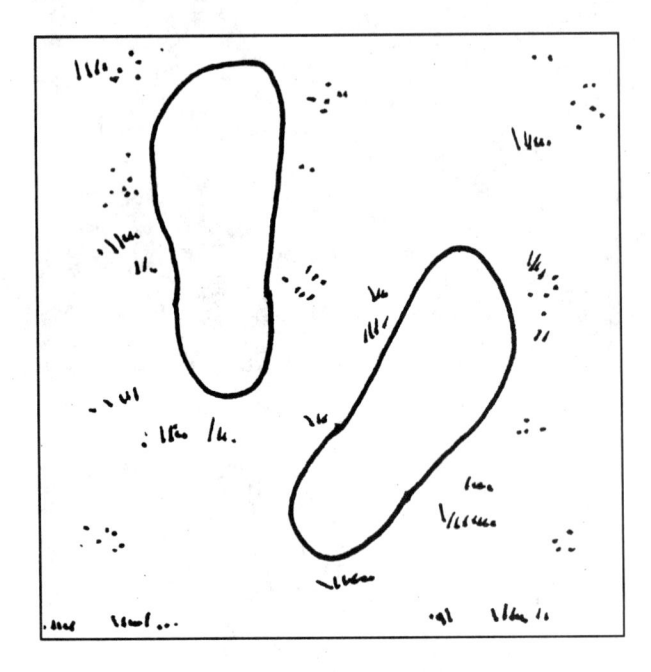

## Snap-Nocks

Snap-nocks are now standard on most modern arrows. For all shooters using any type of mechanical bow string release aid, they're a necessity to eliminate the problem of the arrow coming off the string while at full draw. New finger shooters have similar problems until they are comfortable with the technique. Bowhunters find the snap-nock invaluable for keeping the arrow on the string while sitting in a stand. Students with limited use of their fingers will find that the snap-nocks will cure the problem of the arrow slipping off the string. Many snap-nocks have a small bump on the side of the nock to act as an index indicator so the shooter knows, without looking, which feather or vane faces away from the bow. This is especially helpful to students with visual disabilities or hunters and shooters who want to keep their attention focused on the target.

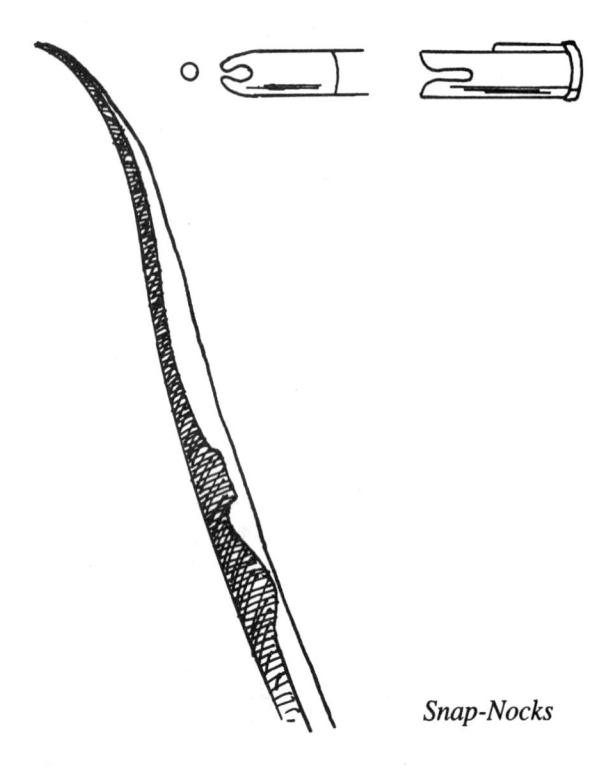

*Snap-Nocks*

*54 Archery Theory & Assistive Devices*

## Nocking Points or Release Cushion Buttons

All shooters, no matter what their abilities, need to use some form of nocking point. They act as a nock locator to insure that each arrow is loaded at the same point on the string. They also eliminate arrows sliping off the bowstring or sliding up and down on the string while loading or at full draw. A nocking point can be as simple as a piece of tape, shrink wrap, tied thread, or a crimped-on brass clamp.

## Cresting Made of Tape

People with visual disabilities are often unable to see the color or pattern of arrow cresting. By using cresting made from particular combination of tape, shooters with visual impairments will be able to identify their arrows from among several similar ones in a target.

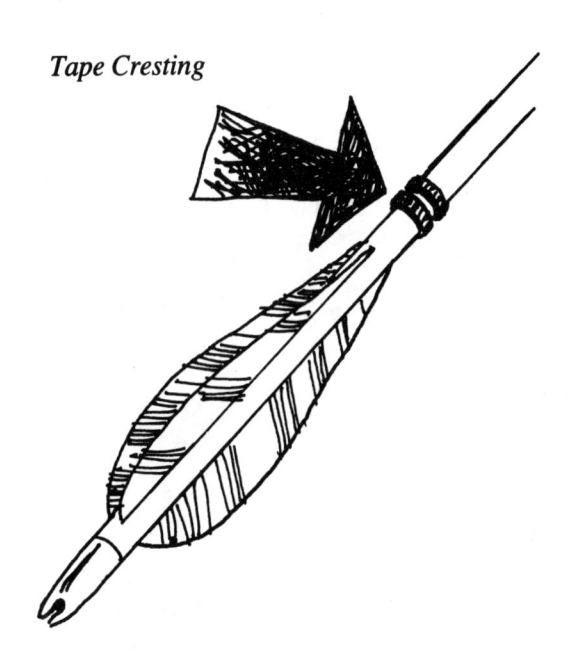

*Tape Cresting*

## Draw-length Ruler

Checking the archer's draw length is usually handled at the archery proshop when they buy their bow. But, if the instructor provides equipment, match the equipment to the shooter. An extra-long arrow with inch-marks along the side of the shaft will make an excellent tool for measuring students' proper draw length. The student simply pulls the arrow to full draw, and the instructor reads off the proper length.

## Feelable Scoring Rings

In order for people with visual disabilities to score their targets, tape bands of string onto the target outlining the scoring areas. Building targets with scoring rings made out of different fabrics such as burlap, linen, or tin foil, also allows the shooter to score the target by touch, rather than by sight.

## Four-fletched Arrows

Archers with sight impairments or learning disabilities often have trouble distinguishing the index feather or vane (generally the different colored feather or vane, that is nocked facing away from the side of the bow) from the other two fletches. A four-fletch arrow is designed not to have an index feather or vane which would eliminate the confusion of proper nocking configuration.

## Flu-Flu Arrows

Flu-Flu arrows, because of their extremely short flying distance, are intended for archery golf, aerial or moving targets. The fletching on a Flu-Flu arrow has not been trimmed as on a traditional arrow. They are made with six or four untrimmed feather fletches, or one full-length untrimmed feather twisted down the shaft. Because they make more noise in flight, are slower and more visable, these may be useful in very early training or while playing games. They are not recommend for serious target training.

## Crossbows

For certain persons with disabilities, the crossbow may be their only avenue to enjoying the shooting sports. Unfortunately, many jurisdictions have regulations either banning or restricting the use of crossbows, so check local laws before using one. Quadriplegics with very little or no arm function can use a crossbow by mounting one in an SR-77 gunrest as mentioned under "Rifle/airgun theory and devices," page 25. Although crossbow cocking devices are available to simplify the process, cocking still requires considerable upper body strength. For persons without that strength or without the aid of another person to do the cocking, a crossbow is impractical. Horton Crossbow Manufacturing Company introduced an electronic cocking device in 1992 to permit persons with physical limitations to use crossbows.

A total of 36 states and five provinces consider crossbows as legal hunting equipment. Eighteen states permit physician certified persons with disabilities to use a crossbow during the state's general archery season.

**Instructor's note:** The following two adaptations should be used only if no other method is acceptable.

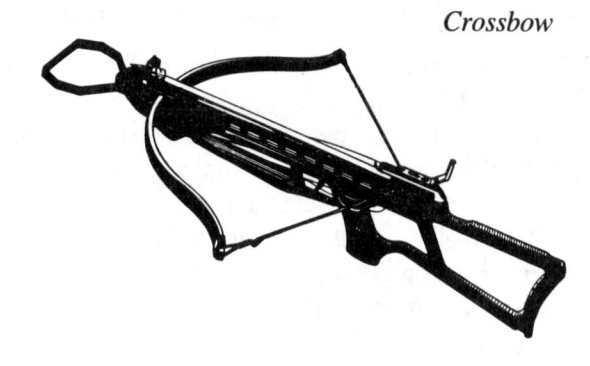

*Crossbow*

## Footbows

A footbow, such as those used for flight shooting, will work for shooters with functioning legs but requires the ability to draw the bowstring. A standard bow can be converted to a footbow if the foot attachment can be perfected.

## Bows Placed Sideways

Rather than use a crossbow, building or buying a system to hold a bow in place horizontally in front of an archer will allow people with cerebral palsy to shoot. People who are missing an arm, hemiplegic, or even missing both arms can shoot with this stand, the last with a teeth tether. A bench press lends itself to quick conversion. Just tape the bow to the uprights.

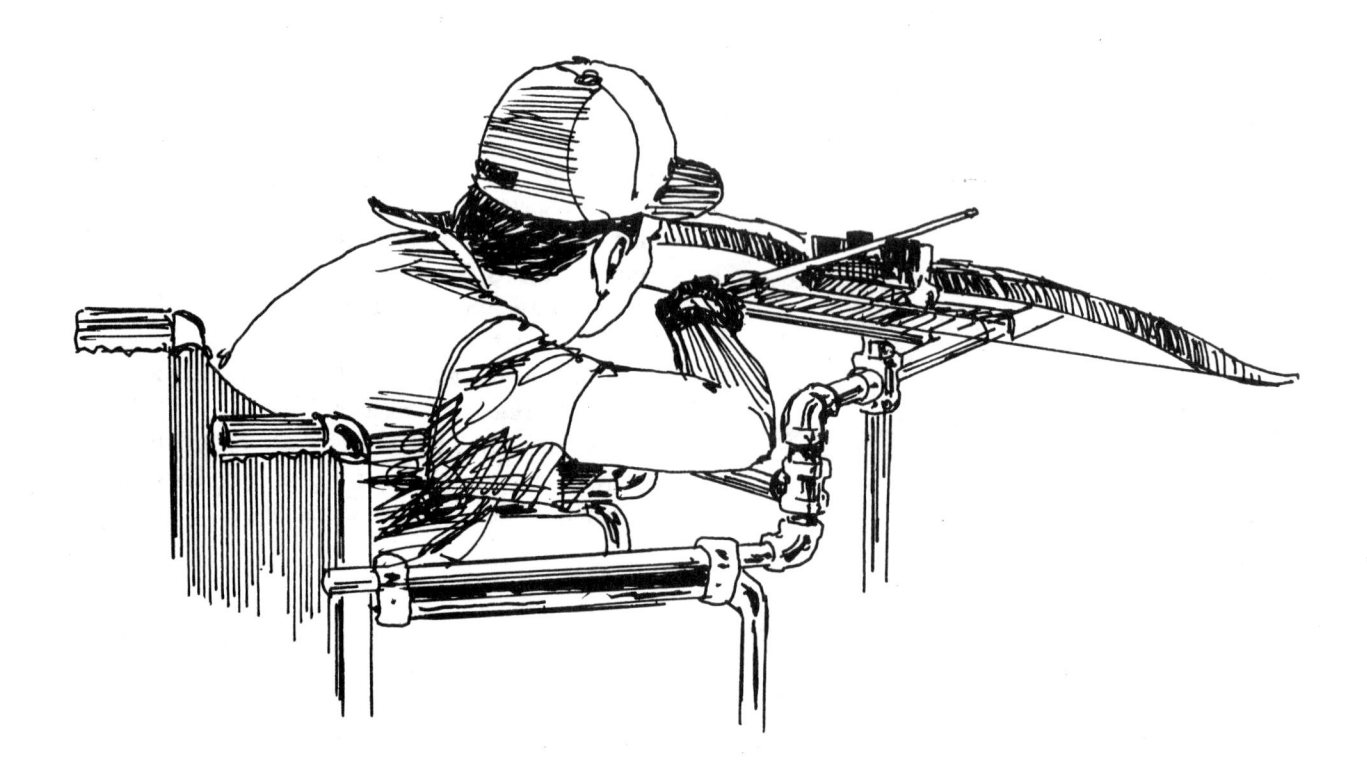

# Archery Lesson Plans

*(Each lesson plan in this book is complete and made to stand alone. You may find duplication in certain parts of each lesson.)*

**Materials needed:**
- Lightweight, low draw-weight compound bows (10-25 lb.)
- One lightweight crossbow
- Arrows — spined, in assorted lengths
- Crossbow bolts to match and Flu-Flu and four-fletch arrows
- Archery targets (10 ring and assorted)
- Balloons
- Clothespins
- Extra bowstrings
- Bow stringers for traditional bows
- Compound bowstringers for changing string
- Carpet squares (see adaptive equipment)
- Sunscreen (if appropriate)
- Insect repellant (if appropriate)
- Drinking cups
- Water cooler
- Bow rack
- Repair tools
- Finger tabs and arm guards
- Several shooting gloves
- Assorted mechanical bowstring release aids
- Masking tape
- Staple guns and staples
- Whistle or bull horn
- First aid kit
- Tissues.

## Motivation and Introduction

The bow and arrow are two of the oldest tools known to mankind, dating back to the Stone Age. As the bow and arrow became dominant, history began to change. Creating lore and legends of Attila, King of the Huns, Genghis Khan, Robin Hood and William Tell, the bow and arrow literally changed the world.

Modern American archery history began in 1828 with the first organized recreational archery club formed in Philadelphia, growing to the over six million archers of today.

Archery adapts easily to individual physical needs. Participants can choose the type of bow they wish to shoot, the style of shooting (i.e. target, field, 3-D, etc.), shooting indoors or outdoors or if they wish to hunt. Archers face the challenge of improving their own score, competing against others or testing their hunting skills in pursuit of wild game.

Excellent physical condition is not required for beginning archery classes. Upper body, shoulder, and arm strength can be developed, as can hand-eye coordination, and both gross and fine motor skills.

**Instructor's notes:** For the student, competitive shooting matches provide an opportunity to both compete against one's self and to share in personal achievements, team spirit, and team pride in competition with others. Participating with a team can create feelings of unity between students and their peers and allows students to develop disciplined self-control.

As hunters and outdoor enthusiasts, the students' knowledge of shooting can enhance their enjoyment of the outdoors thanks to the many options that shooting presents.

However, all students who participate in hunter education and shooting sports programs must learn to handle firearms safely and to practice safety in the field. When teaching any group, cover all aspects of safety thoroughly, including the careful handling of firearms in the home.

**Instructor Role/Activity and Objectives**
1. Give a brief introduction and history of the sport of archery.
2. Explain different types of archery (i.e. bowhunting, targets, filed, 3-D).
3. Show the students the bow and arrow and explain each part.
4. Determine dominant eye.
5. Demonstrate shooting the bow.
6. Describe bow handling and safety.
7. Name the three rules of shooting safety.
8. Explain marksmenship, which combines all of the above skills.
9. Explain the importance of eye protection.

**Student Role/Activity**
1. Students understand how old archery is and that there are different forms of archery to enjoy.
2. Students learn the archery vocabulary and nomenclature.
3. Students see the "shooting sequence" for the first time and begin to mimic the sequence.
4. Students demonstrate skills learned up to this point.
5. Students test each other for dominant eye and with the cutout sight, demonstrate understanding.
6. Students share with other students the application of the three rules.
7. Students try on different eye protection devices.

**Conclusion:** At the end of this lesson each student should:
1. Have spent most of the lesson shooting.
2. Leave with a good feeling about archery.
A. Review
   1. Safety
   2. Individual shooting form
   3. Parts of a bow and arrow.

B. Shooting
   1. Allow the students to choose what they will do that day, i.e. shoot at bull's-eyes, animal targets, or have a tournament.
C. Collect equipment and say farewell.
D. Evaluation of the program by the staff.

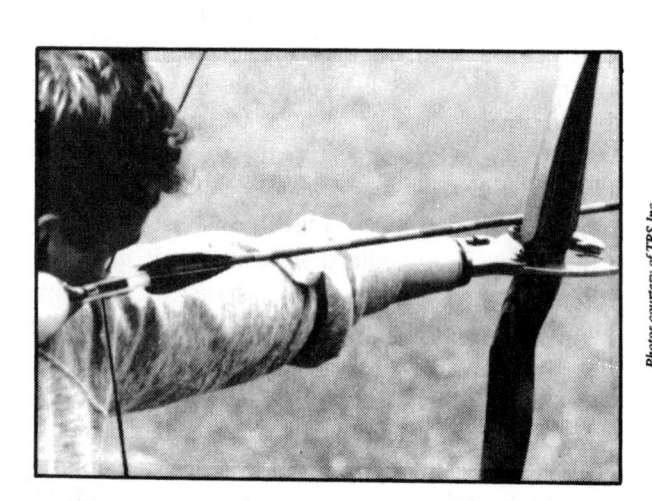

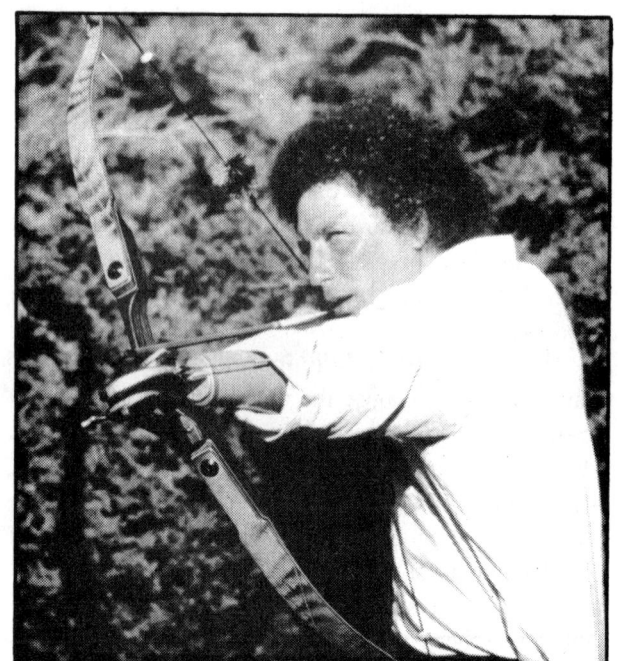

*Photos courtesy of TRS Inc.*

58  *Archery Theory & Assistive Devices*

# Sample Outline

A sample outline for an archery skills program that includes students with disabilities appears below. Modify the outline to fit your particular needs.

### I. Introduction and safety.
At the end of this lesson each student should:
1. Understand archery safety.
2. Begin learning the history of archery.
3. Begin learning archery vocabulary.
4. Be able to identify different parts of a bow and arrow.
   - **A. Introduction of staff and students.**
   - **B. Archery safety.**
      1. Introduce the rules of safe archery:
         a. Never nock an arrow until ready to shoot.
         b. Be sure of your target and what lies beyond.
         c. Treat a bow as you would any firearm.
         d. Keep arrows pointed in a safe direction.
         e. Never dry fire a bow.
         f. Know the range commands.
      2. Explain arrow control. Unlike the rifle, shotgun or pistol, a bow has no muzzle in the traditional sense. But, as the arrow becomes nocked on the bowstring, it becomes the same as a muzzle.
         a. Control is never pointing an arrow at anything you don't want to shoot.
         b. For your safety and the safety of other shooters, never walk around with an arrow nocked on the string.
      3. Show examples of each piece of equipment used.
         a. Bows (longbow, recurve and compound).
         b. Bowstrings and techniques for stringing recurves and longbows.
         c. Arrows.
         d. Armguard and fingertab.
      4. Have students identify each.

**Instructor's note:** Allow students to touch or examine each part.

   5. Explain the function of each piece. Demonstrate how armguards, etc., are worn.
   6. Explain the different kinds of arrows, their differences, and how they are used.
      a. Target arrows (aluminum and carbon).
      b. Small game hunting arrows (Flu-Flu, arrows with blunts and field points).
      c. Big game hunting arrows (show an assortment of legal broadheads).
   7. Shooting form.
      a. Demonstrate a shot, breaking down each part of the shooting sequence.
      b. Without using equipment, have each student mimic each part of the sequence, explaining what they are doing and why.

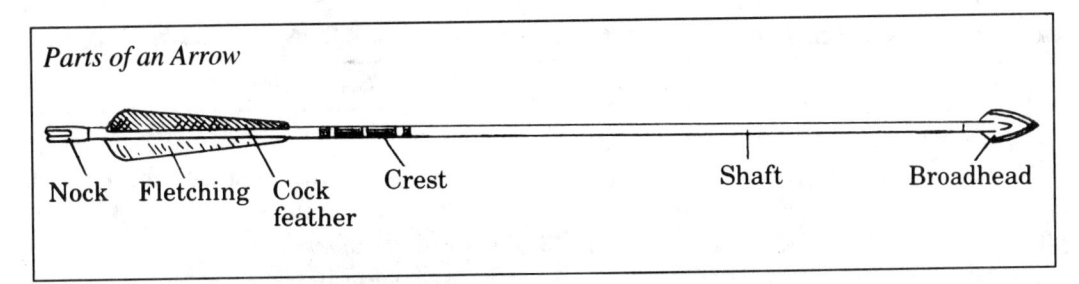

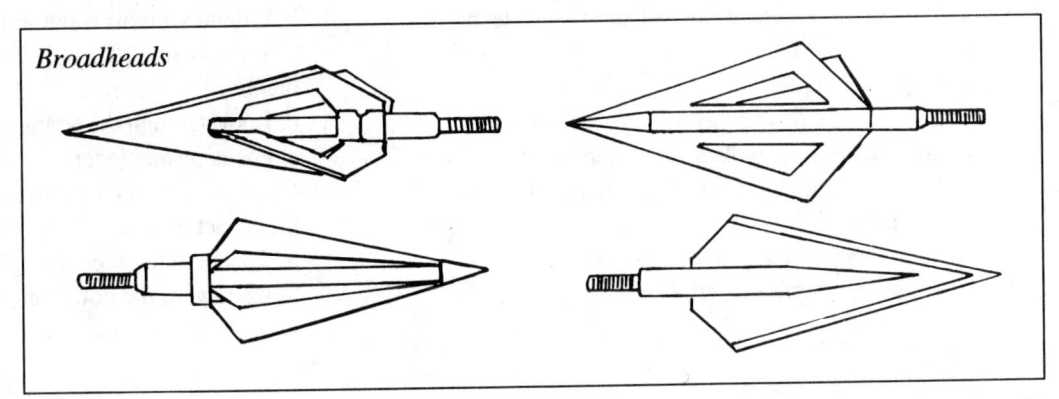

*Parts of an Arrow*

Nock  Fletching  Cock feather  Crest  Shaft  Broadhead

*Broadheads*

## II. Learning the basics.

In this lesson each student should:
1. Review the safety rules.
2. Determine their dominant eye.
3. Learn to use a fingertab and armguard.
4. Determine what length arrows they should shoot.
5. Shoot one or two arrows as time allows.

### A. Equipment review.

Have students repeat the names for each piece of equipment and tell how each is used.

**Instructor's note:** People with hearing, speech, or vision impairments may respond to questions in different ways. "Is this one of the limbs?" combined with handing them the object or writing the question on the board (as appropriate) will be understood by many more students than just saying "Which part is the limb?" Knowing the "signs" (international sign language) for each of the parts will also be helpful.

### B. Safety review.
1. Review the safety rules (page 31), explaining why each is important.
2. Ask questions to confirm understanding.

### C. Determine dominant eye, or the eye the shooter will be using.

(Shooters prefer, if possible, to shoot with their dominant eye. But, if because of a disability that makes it impossible, adjustments and adaptive devices can be used. The following section is for those shooters who will be shooting with their dominant eye.)

The side of the body a given shooter shoots with is determined by their master eye, not by if they are right- or left-handed. Some students will be cross-dominant: right-handed but left-eyed. Teach them to shoot according to their eyes, not their hand, if at all possible.

To determine dominant eye, use one of two techniques:

1. Paper technique.
   a. Hold a piece of paper with a ½" diameter hole cut in the middle at arm's length.
   b. Look through the hole in the paper at an object far away.
   c. Slowly pull the paper back to your face while looking through the hole.
   d. As the hole reaches your face, the hole will surround the dominant eye.

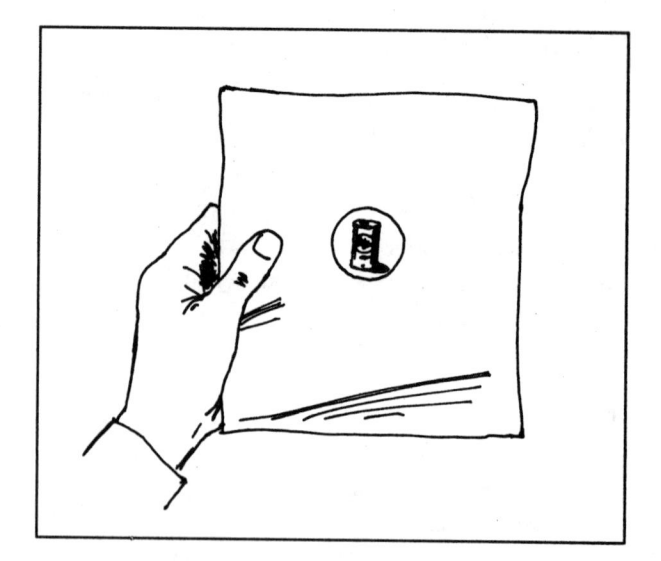

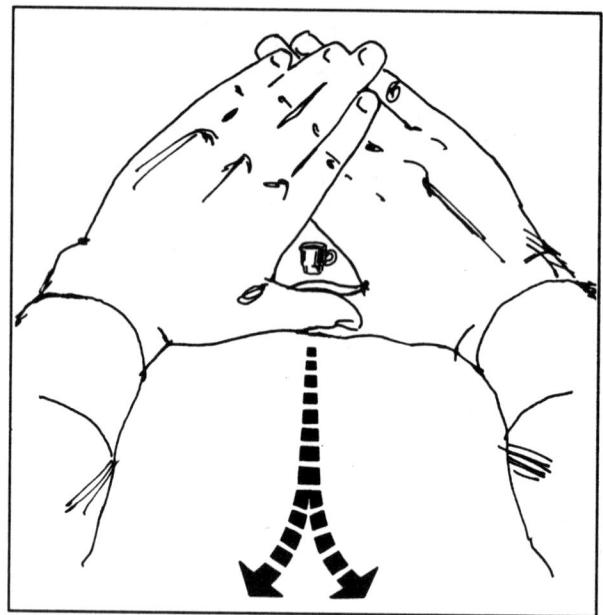

2. Two-hands technique.
   a. Face an object 10 feet away.
   b. Extend your arms out in front of you.
   c. Form a small triangle by overlapping your hands.
   d. Look through the triangle with both eyes.
   e. Focus on an object.
   f. Bring your hands toward your eyes, keeping the object in focus at all times.
   g. To keep the object in sight, the triangle will move toward the dominant eye.

60 *Archery Theory & Assistive Devices*

3. Closing or winking one eye.
   a. Leaving both eyes open leads to better shooting.
   b. Some people see two targets when they leave both eyes open.
   c. To solve the problem have the shooter close one eye or use a blinder of some sort.
4. Arrow length.
   a. Using a lightweight bow, have each student draw an overlength arrow to full draw.
   b. If you are using a measuring arrow, read off the next number ahead of the arrow rest. If not, mark the arrow one inch ahead of the arrow rest and measure to the mark.
   c. Have the students record their proper arrow length.
5. Assign equipment.
   a. Assign each student an armguard, finger tab or glove, quiver, and a compound bow.
   b. Explain how to put the various pieces of equipment on, and assist those who need help.
   c. Review finger tab use and proper anchor and release.
   d. For classroom practice, decide which direction would be safest and announce which wall will be considered downrange. For on-the-range practice, still point out the area that is considered "downrange."
6. Place students on the line and assign "targets."
7. Check the students' clothing, etc. for string clearance.
8. Have the students set their bows down.

**D. Demonstration and class activity.**
1. Demonstrate the steps for shooting, both with and without the string back. Exaggerate each action, including follow through.
2. Students on the line should mimic the instructor's actions.
   a. Don't use arrows!
   b. Have each student visualize what the shot would look like.
   c. Walk up and down the firing line, checking their form.

**Instructor's note:** If a student's elbows bend close to the path of the string, even with proper form, be sure they get an extended armguard.

3. Rotate students and repeat, as necessary. If time allows, move to the range and let students fire their first few shots as detailed in the following lesson.

**E. Gather equipment.**

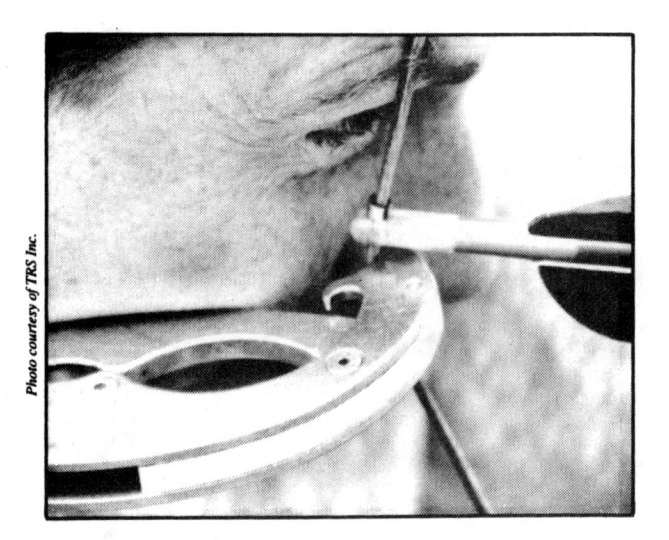

*Photo courtesy of TRS Inc.*

Archery Theory & Assistive Devices

### III. Firing the first shots.
At the end of this lesson each student should:
1. Have a working knowledge of range procedure.
2. Have fired several rounds of arrows.
3. Understand how to safely remove arrows from a target.

#### A. Safety.
1. Review safety rules.
2. Issue equipment, including compound bow, finger tab, armguard and six arrows.

**Instructor's note:** If using recurve bows, teach bow stringing only after the student becomes familiar with the bow and they can physically handle the procedure. Using a bowstringer is necessary to prolong the life of a recurve bow, but for someone lacking the knowledge or strength, it can be dangerous. If using recurves, have stringers available and if the students are able, teach them to properly use a bowstringer. Emphasize bending the bow limbs *evenly* as it is being strung.

#### B. Eye protection.
1. Explain the hows and whys of eye protection.
2. Demonstrate how each type is worn.
Allow students to handle the different types.

**Instructor's note:** Students with visual impairments still need eye protection! In addition to being sensory organs, eyes are soft and easily damaged. Protect their senses - have them wear eye protection.

#### C. Using a bowstringer.
1. Place the bow face (the side of the bow that faces the archer while shooting) on the ground with the string looped over each limb.
2. Place the bowstringer's caps over either tip of the bow and step on the stringer.
3. Lift on the bow riser until the limbs are bent to be able to slip the string into place.
4. Relax the bowstringer slowly, checking that the string is well seated in its notches.

**Instructor's Note:** Use of a bowstringer to string a recurve bow requires the user's ability to draw and hold the bow at its maximum weight.

#### D. Assign each student a target.
#### E. Live fire.
1. Review anchor, string alignment and/or string peep, pin sight and nocking point.
2. Talk the students through the first six shots.
3. Discuss the proper way to approach the target.
4. Give the signal to retrieve, (two whistles, voice, lights or flags).

**Instructor's note:** The next exercise is on removing arrows from the target. Help may be needed in this process, depending on the mobility of the shooter, the degree of assistive devices used, and if the devices can be removed easily.

**F. Demonstrate how to safely remove arrows from the target.**
   1. Check that no one is behind you.
   2. Place a hand on the target face to keep the backstop from falling over.
   3. Pull the arrow from the target using an unscrewing motion.
   4. Emphasize standing to the side to avoid being struck by a nock when someone else pulls their arrow free.
   5. Demonstrate when to pull an arrow through a target.
   6. Check to see if the feathers have entered the target.
   7. Describe how pulling an arrow from within the target will damage the feathers on an arrow, even if the feathers have only passed partially into the target.

**G. Repeat as time allows.**
**H. Equipment check-in.**
**I. Evaluation.**
   1. Note whether the safety rules were followed.
   2. Recognize the successes of each student.

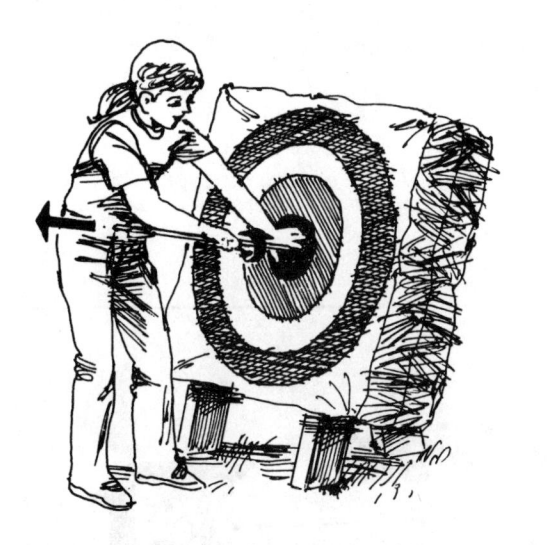

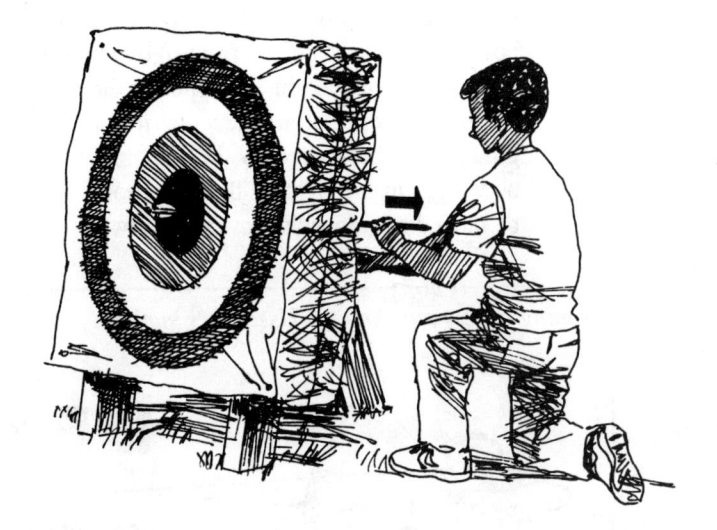

**IV. A day of shooting.**
At the end of this lesson each student should:
1. Have fired several rounds of arrows.
2. Have a better understanding of anchor, release, etc.
3. Understand how to score an indoor FITA target.
4. Understand how a pin-style bowsight works.
   **A. Demonstration of sights.**
   1. Gather the students together.
   2. Demonstrate the use of a bowsight.
      a. Explain how they work by holding an oversize cardboard cut-out of a bowsight at arm's length against the riser of a bow.
      b. Raise and lower the bow and sight against a fixed point on a wall or post.
      c. Show how the height of the bow changes depending on which pin you use.
      d. Explain other types of bow sights including single and multiple cross hairs, scopes and lasers.
      e. Explain that bow sights are adjusted. The bow sight is the same as a front sight on a rifle and must be moved in the opposite direction to change point of impact; i.e. if the shot group is to be moved to the left, move the bow sight to the right; if the shot group is to be moved up, move the bow sight down.

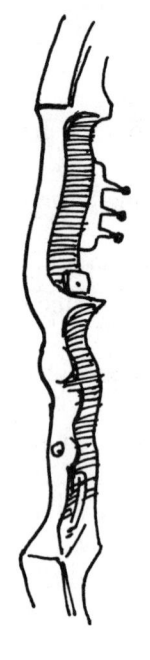

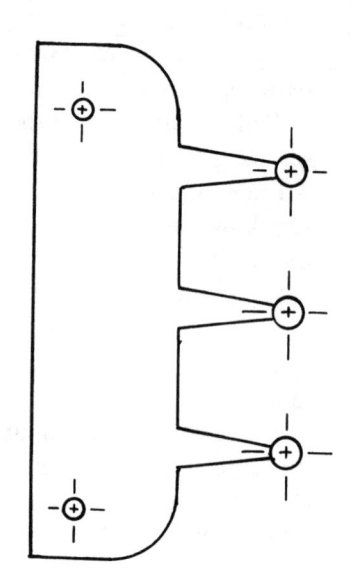

*Pin-sight Cut-outs*

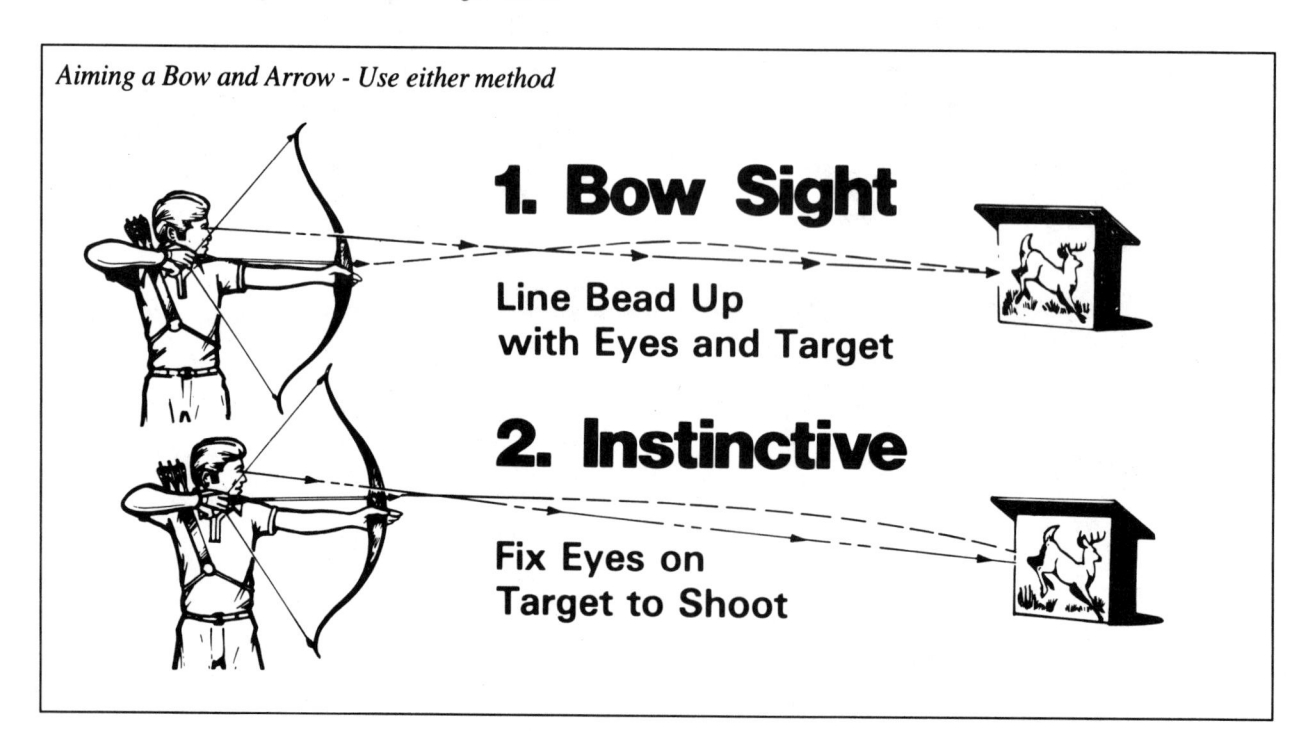

*Aiming a Bow and Arrow - Use either method*

**1. Bow Sight**
Line Bead Up with Eyes and Target

**2. Instinctive**
Fix Eyes on Target to Shoot

*64  Archery Theory & Assistive Devices*

## V. Shooting games.

At the end of this lesson, each student should:

1. Have reviewed the material covered in class to date.
2. Have been introduced to alternative targets (3-D, FITA, Spot, Hunter, etc.).
3. Have played Team Tic-Tac-Toe using balloons.

### A. Review discussion.
1. Review and ask questions about the material covered in the first four lessons.
2. Emphasize safety.

### B. Team Tic-Tac-Toe.
1. Divide the class in half and have each student blow up two balloons each, if possible, as while issuing equipment and explaining the rules.
2. Arrange two 3 by 3 grids of balloons, one for each team.
3. Arrange the teams in single-file rows, facing the target.
4. Shooters fire one shot per shooter each team, one side, then the other, each trying to pop three balloons in a row.
5. Play the game two out of three, or three out of five as time allows.

### C. Go through other targets and explain scoring.
1. Set up each target butt with a different target face.
2. Have the students rotate from one target to the next, shooting three arrows at each. While they are doing this, impress upon them that each target takes the same concentration and that they should pick the spot in the center of the bull's-eye and shoot at that only.
3. Give them the chance to shoot at each type of target face.

## VI. Evaluate and clean-up.
### A. Were the safety procedures followed?
### B. Is the range clean?
### C. Did everyone have fun?
### D. Is all the equipment in?

## VII. Evaluation of lessons.

# Appendix I
## Uniform Federal Assessibility Standards

This document presents uniform standards for the design, construction, and alteration of buildings so that physically handicapped persons will have ready access to and use of them in accordance with the Architectural Barriers Act, 42 U.S.C. 4151-4157.

**For further information contact:**
General Services Administration
18th and F Streets N.W., Room 3044
Washington, D.C. 20405
(202) 566-0038

Department of Defense, Office of the
Deputy Assistant Secretary of Defense
(Equal Opportunity), Room 3E317
The Pentagon, Washington, D.C. 20301
(202) 697-8661

Department of Housing and
Urban Development
451 7th Street S.W., Room 9220
Washington, D.C. 20410
(202) 755-6454

Real Estate and
Buildings Department
U.S. Postal Service
475 L'Enfant Plaza West S.W.
Washington, D.C. 20260-6424
(202) 268-3139

For TDD communication,
call (202) 426-6030.
These are not toll-free numbers.

---

The United States Equal Employment Opportunity Commission and the United States Department of Justice have jointly produced the **Americans with Disabilities Act Handbook**. This comprehensive publication provides background, summary, rule-making history, overview of the regulations, section-by-section analysis of comments and revisions, P.L. 101-336 and annotated regulations of Titles I, II, and III, plus appendices and related federal disability laws. One copy free upon request from EEOC or DOJ, or from the Disability and Business Technical Assistance Centers. Multiple copies can be purchased from:

U.S. Government Printing Office
Superintendent of Documents
Mail Stop: SSOP
Washington, DC 20402-9328
(202) 783-3238 voice
(202) 512-1426 TDD

---

Always check state, provincial and local regulations, which are subject to change, even on emergency notice. In addition, be certain to check for correct addresses and telephone numbers, as they can also change from what appears in this manual.

# Appendix II
## Assessibility Checklist

**Parking Lots**
1. Are accessible spaces provided? Are they marked?
2. Is there adequate space for people in wheelchairs or on braces to get in or out onto a level surface? (Approximately 60 inches clearance).

**Walks**
1. Are the walkways at least 48 inches wide? Is the gradient not more than 5 percent?
2. Are they smooth? No steps or abrupt changes in level?
3. Are they firm enough that wheelchairs can get adequate traction?
4. Where they cross, do they blend to a common level?
5. Is there room around doorways, etc. for someone in a wheelchair to sit level and negotiate the door?

**Ramps**
1. Do the ramps have handrails on at least one side? The rails should be 32 inches from the floor, smooth, and extend at least 1 foot beyond either side of the ramp.
2. Are the ramps non-skid?
3. Are there 6 feet of level runway at the bottom of each?
4. On long ramps, is there a place to rest?

**Entrances/Exits**
1. Is at least one main entrance usable by someone in a wheelchair?
2. Can people in wheelchairs get to the elevators?

**Doors and Doorways**
1. Are the openings in the doors at least 32 inches wide?
2. Could a very weak person open and control the doors?

3. Is the floor on either side of the door level for 5 feet?
4. Are there bumps at the doorsills that might cause problems?

**Stairs and Steps**
1. Are there handrails 32 inches from the floor on at least one side?
2. Is there a handrail that extends at least 18 inches beyond the steps?

**Floors**
1. Non-skid?
2. Are all the levels on each floor accessible by ramp?

**Rest Rooms**
1. One per gender?
2. Can physically handicapped people use them?
3. Can someone in a wheelchair turn around (needs a 60 by 60 inch space).
4. Do toilet rooms have at least one stall that:
   a. is 5 feet wide?
   b. is at least 5 feet deep?
   c. has a 32 inch wide door that swings out?
   d. has grab bars on each side, 33 inches high, parallel to the floor that a person could support themselves on (1 1/2 inches in diameter with 1 1/2 inches of clearance to the wall)?
   e. has at least 48 inches between the toilet and the stall entrance?
5. Is there a urinal 19 inches from the floor?
6. Is there a towel no higher than 40 inches from the floor?
7. Are racks, dispensers, and disposal units located to the side and within reach, rather than directly above?
8. Mirror no higher than 40 inches.

**Water Fountains**
1. Is there one?
2. Can a person with a physical disability use it?
3. Can a person with a physical disability reach it?
4. Are the controls up front, or do you have to reach?
5. Can a person in a wheelchair use and operate the fountain?

**Public Telephones**
1. Is the height of the dial less than 48 inches from the floor?
2. How about the coin slot?
3. Are there marked telephones that can accommodate hearing impairments?

**Elevators**
1. If there is more than one story in a building, is there a wheelchair-accessible elevator?
2. Are all controls less than 48 inches from the floor?
3. Are buttons labeled with raised lettering?
4. Are they easy to push?
5. Is the cab at least 5 feet by 5 feet?

**Controls**
1. Are all fire alarms, drapery cords, etc. within reach of people in wheelchairs?

**Hazards**
1. Are there low-hanging signs, lights, or fixtures (minimum 7 feet from the floor)?
2. Is the lighting adequate, especially on ramps?
3. Are exit signs easily identifiable to all people, including those with disabilities?

**Other Features**
1. Is there a hard-packed, wooden, or paved trail to ranges, club houses, parking lots?
2. Does your range/classroom have accessible parking spaces?
3. Can someone in a wheelchair get their chair under the overhangs of a table?

# Appendix III

## Hunter Education Administrators
### Coordinators of Hunter Education Programs in the states and provinces

**ALABAMA**
Hunter Safety Administrator
Game & Fish Div.
64 N. Union Street
Montgomery, AL 36104
205/242-3623

**ALASKA**
Hunter Safety Administrator
Div. of Game & Fish
333 Raspberry Rd.
Anchorage, AK 99518-1599
907/267-2187

**ALBERTA**
Hunter Education Administrator
Fish & Wildlife Division
Petroleum Plaza
9945 108 Street
Edmonton, Alberta T5K 2G6
403/427-6735

**ARIZONA**
Hunter Education Administrator
Arizona Game & Fish Dept.
2222 West Greenway Rd.
Phoenix, AZ 85023
602/789-3241

**ARKANSAS**
Hunter Education Administrator
Arkansas Game & Fish Comm.
#2 Natural Resources Dr.
Little Rock, AR 72205
501/223-6414

**BRITISH COLUMBIA**
Recreation Education Administrator
Ministry of Environment/Wildlife Br.
780 Blanshard St.
Victoria, B.C. V8V 1X5
604/387-9760

**CALIFORNIA**
Hunter Safety Training Officer
Dept. of Fish & Game
1416 9th St. Room 1342-1
Sacramento, CA 95814
(916) 653-9727

**COLORADO**
Hunter Safety Administrator
Div. of Wildlife
6060 Broadway
Denver, CO 80216
303/291-7264

**CONNECTICUT**
Hunter Education Administrator
Franklin Wildlife Mngmt. Area
391 Route 32
North Franklin, CT 06254
203/642-7239

**DELAWARE**
Hunter Education Administrator
Div. of Fish & Wildlife
89 Kings Way
Dover, DE 19903
302/739-3486

**FLORIDA**
Hunter Education Administrator
Game & Fresh Water Fish Comm.
Farris Bryant Bldg.
620 South Meridian St.
Tallahassee, FL 32399-1600
904/488-4676

**GEORGIA**
Hunter Education Administrator
Law Enforcement
2070 US Highway 278, SE
Social Circle, GA 30279
404/918-6409

### HAWAII
Conservation Education Program Specialist
Dept. of Land & Natural Resources
1130 N. Nimitz Highway #B-299
Honolulu, HI 96817-4521
808/587-0200 or -0206

### IDAHO
Hunter Education Administrator
Fish & Game Dept.
600 S. Walnut St., Box 25
Boise, ID 83707
208/334-2633

### ILLINOIS
Safety Education Administrator
Illinois Dept. of Conservation
524 S. 2nd Street
Springfield, IL 62701-1787
217/782-6431

### INDIANA
Outdoor Education Officer
Dept. of Natural Resources
402 W Washington St W-255D
Indianapolis, IN 46204
317/232-4010

### IOWA
Recreational Safety Administrator
Dept. of Natural Resources
Wallace State Office Bldg.
Des Moines, IA 50319-0034
515/281-8652

### KANSAS
Wildlife Education Administrator
Kansas Dept. of Wildlife & Parks
512 SE 25th Avenue
Pratt, KS 67124
316/672-5911

### KENTUCKY
Dept. of Fish & Wildlife
Information & Education Div.
#1 Game Farm Rd.
Frankfort, KY 40601
502/564-4762

### LOUISIANA
Dept. of Wildlife Fisheries
P.O. Box 278
U.S. Hwy 71 N (for Fed Ex)
Tioga LA 71477
318/487-5885

### MAINE
Safety Officer
Dept. of Inland Fisheries & Wildlife
284 State St., Station 41
Augusta, ME 04333
207/287-5220

### MANITOBA
Hunter Safety Administrator
Dept. of Natural Resources
1495 St. James Street #200
Winnipeg, Manitoba R3H 4W9
204/945-6646

**MARYLAND**
Outdoor Education Director
MD Natural Resources Police
69 Prince George Street
Annapolis, MD 21401
410/974-2327

**MASSACHUSETTS**
Hunter Education Administrator
Hunter Education Program
Division of Law Enforcement
P.O. Box 408
Westminister, MA 01473-0408
508/792-7434

**MICHIGAN**
Supervisor of Recr. Safety Education
Dept. of Natural Resources
530 W. Allegan
Lansing, MI 48933
517/335-3410

**MINNESOTA**
Hunter Safety Administrator
Dept. of Natural Resources
500 Lafayette Rd. Box 47
St. Paul, MN 55155-4047
612/296-0655

**MISSISSIPPI**
Hunter Education Administrator
Dept. of Wildlife, Fisheries & Parks
P.O. Box 451
Jackson, MS 39205
601/364-2190

**MISSOURI**
Hunter Safety Administrator
Dept. of Conservation
2901 W. Truman Blvd.
Jefferson City, MO 65102-0180
314/751-4115

**MONTANA**
Hunter Education Administrator
Dept. of Fish Wildlife & Parks
1420 E. Sixth Ave.
Helena, MT 59620
406/444-4046

**NEBRASKA**
Hunter Safety Administrator
Game & Parks Comm.
P.O. Box 30370
Lincoln, NE 68503
402/471-5434

**NEVADA**
Hunter Safety Administrator
Dept. of Wildlife
P.O. Box 10678
Reno, NV 89520
702/688-1500

**NEW BRUNSWICK**
Hunter Safety Administrator
Dept. of Natural Resources & Energy
P.O. Box 6000
Fredericton, NB E3B 5H1
506/453-2440

NEWFOUNDLAND
Hunter Education Administrator
Wildlife Division
Bldg 810 Pleasantville/PO Box 8700
St. Johns, Newfoundland A1B 4J6
709/729-2549

NEW HAMPSHIRE
Hunter Education Administrator
Fish & Game Dept.
2 Hazen Dr.
Concord, NH 03301
603/271-3212

NEW JERSEY
Hunter Education Administrator
NJ Div. of Fish, Game, & Wildlife
CN 400
Trenton, NJ 08625
609/629-0552

NEW MEXICO
Hunting Training Administrator
Dept. of Game & Fish
3841 Midway Place N.E.
Albuquerque, NM 87109
505/841-8881 ext. 919

NEW YORK
Sportsman Ed. Administrator
Dept. of Environmental Conserv.
Div. of Fish & Wildlife
50 Wolf Rd., Room 122
Albany, NY 12233-4800
518/457-2994

NORTH CAROLINA
Hunter Safety Administrator
Wildlife Res. Comm./Enforcement Div.
512 N. Salisbury St.
Raleigh, NC 27604
919/733-7191

NORTH DAKOTA
Hunter Education Supervisor
Game & Fish Dept.
100 N. Bismarck Expressway
Bismarck, ND 58501
701/221-6300 - 6316

NORTHWEST TERRITORIES
Coord. Firearms Safety/Fur Mgmt.
Dept. of Renewable Resources
Government of NWT
Box 1320
Yellowknife, NWT X1A 2L9
403/920-6401

NOVA SCOTIA
Hunter Education Administrator
Dept. of Natural Resources
Enforcement & Hunter Safety
2nd floor, Founder's Square
1701 Hollis St.
Halifax, Nova Scotia B3J 2T9
902/424-5254

OHIO
Outdoor Skills Section
Ohio Division of Wildlife
1840 Belcher Drive
Columbus, OH 43224-1329
614/265-6544

OKLAHOMA
Hunter Education Administrator
Dept. of Wildlife Conservation
1801 North Lincoln
Oklahoma City, OK  73105
405/521-4650

ONTARIO
Hunter Education Administrator
Wildlife Branch
90 Shepherd Ave. East
North York, Ontario M2N 3A1
416/314-1036.

OREGON
Hunter Education Supervisor
Oregon Dept. of Fish & Wldlf.
2501 S.W. 1st Ave.
Portland, OR  97201
503/229-5400

PENNSYLVANIA
Hunter Education Administrator
Game Commission
Hunter-Trapper Educ. Div.
2001 Elmerton Ave.
Harrisburg, PA  17110-9797
717/787-7015

PRINCE EDWARD ISLAND
Conservation Officer
Fish & Wildlife Division
Box 2000
Charlottetown, PEI C1A 7N8
902/368-4683

QUEBEC
Hunter Safety Administrator
Dept. of Leisure, Fish & Game
150th St., Cyrille Blvd.
Quebec City, Quebec  G1R 4Y1
418/644-8371

RHODE ISLAND
State Firearms Safety Administrator
Fish & Wildlife - DEM
Washington County Gov't Center
Tower Hill Rd.
Wakefield, RI  02879
401/789-7055

SASKATCHEWAN
Hunter Education Administrator
Firearms Safety Div.
Dept. of Parks & Renewable Res.
3211 Albert St.
Regina, Saskatchewan  S4S 5W6
306/787-2314

SOUTH CAROLINA
Hunter Safety Administrator
Wildlife & Marine Res. Dept.
Rembert C. Dennis Bldg.
1000 Assembly St., Box 167
Columbia, SC  29202
803/734-4003

SOUTH DAKOTA
Hunter Safety Administrator
Dept. of Game, Fish & Parks
445 E. Capitol, Anderson Bldg.
Pierre, SD  57501
605/773-3630

TENNESSEE
Hunter Education Supervisor
Wildlife Resources Agency
P.O. Box 40747
Nashville, TN 37204
615/781-6538

TEXAS
Conservation Education Supervisor
Parks & Wildlife Dept.
4200 Smith School Road
Austin, TX 78744
512/389-4999

UTAH
Hunter Education Administrator
State of Utah
Div. of Wildlife Resources
1596 West North Temple St.
Salt Lake City, UT 84116
801/538-4725

VERMONT
Hunter Education Administrator
Dept of Fish & Wildlife
103 S. Main Street
Waterbury, VT 05676
802/241-3700

VIRGINIA
Hunter Education Administrator
VA Dept. of Game & Inl. Fish.
Law Enforcement Div.
P.O. Box 11104
Richmond, VA 23230
804/367-1000

WASHINGTON
Hunter Education Administrator
Dept. of Wildlife
215 Thurston Ave.
Olympia, WA 98501-1091
206/753-4476

WEST VIRGINIA
Hunter Safety Administrator
DNR-Law Enforcement Section
Capitol Complex, Bldg. 3
1900 Kanawha Blvd. E.
Charleston, WV 25305
304/558-2783

WISCONSIN
Hunter Education Administrator
Dept. of Natural Resources
P.O. Box 7921
Madison, WI 53707
608/266-1317

WYOMING
Hunter Education Administrator
Game & Fish Department
5400 Bishop Blvd.
Cheyenne, WY 82006
307/777-4538

YUKON
Hunter Education Administrator (R-7)
Dept. of Renewable Resources
Government of Yukon
P.O. Box 2703
Whitehorse, Yukon Y1A 2C6
403/667-5617

# Appendix IV
## U.S. Fish and Wildlife Service Region Offices and Other Federal Agencies
(Caretakers of the U.S. National Wildlife Refuge System)

**Region 1 — CA, ID, HI, OR, WA**
Eastside Federal Complex
911 NE 11th Avenue
Portland, OR 97232-4181
(503) 231-6128

**Region 2 — AZ, NM, OK, TX**
P.O. Box 1306
Albuquerque, NM 87103
(505) 766-2095
(505) 766-2096

**Region 3 — IL, IN, IA, MI, MN, MO, OH, WI**
Federal Building, Fort Snelling
Twin Cities, MN 55111
(612) 725-3596

**Region 4 — AR, AL, FL, GA, KY, LA, MS, NC, SC, TN, PR, VI**
Richard B. Russell Federal Building
1875 Century Blvd, Rm 207
Atlanta, GA 30345
(404) 679-4159

**Region 5 — CT, DE, MA, MD, ME, NH, NJ, NY, PA, RI, VA, VT, WV**
300 Westgate Center Drive
Hadley, MA 01035-9589
(413) 253-8513

**Region 6 — CO, KS, MT, NE, ND, SD, UT, WY**
Box 25486, Denver Federal Center
Denver, Colorado 80225
(303) 236-7392

**Region 7 — AK**
1011 E. Tudor Road
Anchorage, AK 99503
(907) 786-3487

**Department of the Interior**
1849 C Street NW, Rm. 670-ARLSQ
Washington, DC 20240
(703) 358-1744 (Refuge Department)

**U.S. Army Corps of Engineers**
(The following offices hold some form of hunting for persons with disabilities.)

Arkabutla Lake
Rt. 1 Box 572
Coldwater, MS 38618
(601) 562-6261

Grenada Lake
P.O. Box 903
Grenada, MS 38901
(601) 226-5911

Somerville Lake
P.O. Box 549
Somerville, TX 77879
(409) 596-1622

Lake Shelbyville
Rt. 4 Box 128B
Shelbyville, IL 62565

Mark Twain Lake
RR 2 Box 20A
Monroe City, MO 63456
(314) 735-4097

Carlyle Lake
801 Lake
Carlyle, IL 62231
(618) 594-2484

Rend Lake
RR 3
Benton, IL 62812
(618) 724-2493

Tulsa District
P.O. Box 61
Tulsa, OK 74121
(918) 581-7356

# Canadian Provincial and Territorial Wildlife Ministers

**Alberta**
Minister of Environmental Protection (Wildlife)
Government of Alberta
Legislature Building, Room 323
Edmonton, Alberta
T5K 2B6
(403) 427-2391

**British Columbia**
Minister of Environment,
Lands and Parks Government of
British Columbia
Parliament Buildings
Victoria, British Columbia
V8V 1X4
(604) 387-1187

**Manitoba**
Minister of Natural Resources (Wildlife)
Government of Manitoba
Legislative Building, Room 314
450 Broadway Avenue
Winnipeg, Manitoba
R3C 0V8
(204) 945-3730

**New Brunswick**
Minister of Natural Resources
and Energy (Wildlife)
Government of New Brunswick
Post Office Box 6000, Room 312
Hugh John Fleming Forestry Complex
fredericton, New Brunswick
E3B 5H1
(506) 453-2501

**Newfoundland**
Minister of Tourism and Culture (Wildlife)
Government of Newfoundland and Labrador
P.O. Box 8700, 2nd Floor
West Block
St. John's, Newfoundland
A1B 4J6
(709) 729-0657

**Northwest Territories**
Minister of Renewable Resources
(Environment and Wildlife)
Government of Northwest Territories
P.O. Box 1320
Yellowknife, Northwest Territories
X1A 2L9
(403) 873-7128

**Nova Scotia**
Minister of Natural Resources (Wildlife)
Government of Nova Scotia
Founders Square Building
1701 Hollis Street, 2nd Floor
P.O. Box 698
Halifax, Nova Scotia
B3J 2T9
(902) 424-4037

**Ontario**
Minister of Natural Resources (Wildlife)
Government of Ontario
99 Wellesley Street W., 6th Floor
Whitney Block, Queen's Park
Toronto, Ontario
M7A 1W3
(416) 314-2301

**Prince Edward Island**
Minister of Environmental Resources
(Environment and Wildlife)
Government of Prince Edward Island
11 Kent Street
P.O. Box 2000
Charlottetown, Prince Edward Island
C1A 7N8
(902) 368-6410

**Québec**
Ministre du Loisir, de la Chasse et de la Pêche
Gouvernement du Québec
150, boulevard St Cyrille est
17th étage
Québec (Québec)
G1R 4X1
(418) 643-6527

**Saskatchewan**
Minister of the Environment
and Resource Manager (Wildlife)
Government of Saskatchewan
Legislative Building, Room 348
Regina, Saskatchewan
S4S 0B3
(306) 787-0393

**Yukon Territory**
Minister of Renewable Resources
(Environment and Wildlife)
Government of the Yukon Territory
2071 2nd Avenue
P.O. Box 2703
Whitehorse, Yukon Territory
Y1A 2C6
(403) 667-5376

**Canada**
Minister of Environment
House of Commons
Ottawa, Ontario
K1A 0A6
(613) 943-1106

# Appendix V
## National Organizations

Access Oregon
2600 Oregon
Portland, OR 97214

Accessible Journeys
35 West Sellers Ave.
Ridley Park, PA 19078
(215) 521-0339, FAX (215) 521-6959

Alabama Handicapped Sportsmen
44 Huntington Place
Northport, AL 35476

All Outdoors, Inc.
P.O. Box 1100
Redmond, OR 97756

Amateur Trap Association
Vandalia, Ohio
(513) 898-4638

American Wheelchair Archers
Rd. #2, Box 2043
West Sunbury, PA 16061
(412) 735-4359

The Athletic Congress of the United States
P.O. Box 120
Indianapolis, IN 46202
(317) 638-9155

Boy Scouts of America
1325 Walnut Hill Lane
Irving, TX 75038-3096
(214) 580-2000

Canadian Blind Sports Association
333 River Road
Ottawa, Ontario
Canada K1L 8H9

Canadian Wheelchair Sports Association
1600 James Naismith Drive
Gloucester, Ontario
Canada, K1B5N4
(613) 748-5685, FAX (613) 748-5722

Capable Partners (Pairs able-bodied hunters with disabled hunters.)
P.O. Box 47942
Plymouth, MN 55447-0942
(612) 475-1451

Cooperative Wilderness Handicapped Outdoor Group
Idaho State University
Box 8118
Pocatello, ID 83209

Courage Center
3915 Golden Valley Road
Golden Valley, MN 55422

Disabled Outdoor Foundation
320 Lake Street
Oak Park, IL 60302

Disabled Shooting Services
102 Park Ave.
Rockledge, PA 19111
(215) 379-2359

Dwarf Athletic Association of America
3725 West Holmes
Lansing, MI 48910
(517) 393-3116

Environmental Traveling Companions
Building C, Room 360
Fort Mason Center
San Francisco, CA 94123

Excalibur Leisure Skills Center
393 Knowton Ave.
Kenmore, NY 14217

Fishing Has No Boundaries
P.O. Box 175
Hayward, WI 54843

Florida Disabled Outdoors
2213 Tallahassee Drive
Tallahassee, FL 32308

Florida Council of Handicapped
3012 Calumet Drive
Orlando, FL 32810

Four-H, National Council
7100 Connetticut Ave.
Chevy Chase, MD 20815-4999
(301) 961-2800

Future Farmers of America
P.O. Box 15160
National FFA Center
5632 Mount Vernon Highway
Alexandria, VA 22309
(703) 360-3600

Handicapped Boaters Association
P.O. Box 1134 Ansonia Station
New York, NY 10023

Hunter Education Association
P.O. Box 525/865 East 12200
South Draper, UT 84020

The Ice House
14 Beverly Place
Bridgeport, CT 06610

Information Center for Citizens with Disabilities
20 Park Plaza Room 300
Boston, MA 02116

Invitational for Physically Challenged
240 Lynnbrook Drive
Eugene, OR 97404

Lake Merritt's Adapted Boating
Oakland Office of Parks and Recreation
1520 Lakeside Drive
Oakland, CA 94612

National Archery Association of the United States
1750 East Boulder St.
Colorado Springs, CO 80909-5778
(719) 578-4576
Attn: Handicapped Committee, Chairperson

National Bowhunter Education Foundation
P.O. Box 2007
Fond du Lac, WI 54936
(414) 923-5238

National Council on Handicapped
330 C Street N.W.
Suite 3121
Washington, DC 20202

National Easter Seal Society
70 East Lake Street
Chicago, IL 60601
(312-726-6200, (312) 726-4258 TDD,
(312) 726-1494

National Guard Four Position Air Rifle Program
Unit Marksmanship Support Center
Attn: Youth Programs
P.O. Box 17267
Nashville, TN 37217-0267

National Handicapped Sports
and Recreation Association
1145 19th Street Northwest, Suite 717
Washington, DC 20036
(301) 217-0960

National Muzzleloading Rifle Association
1680 Optimist Rd. - Hardin Co.
Lebanon Jct., KY 40150
(502) 737-1163

National Organization on Disability
910 16th Street N.W., Suite 600
Washington, DC 20006

National Rifle Association
11250 Waples Mill Rd.
Fairfax, VA 22030
(703) 267-1000

National Shooting Sports Foundation
Flintlock Ridge Office Center
11 Mile Hill Road
Newtown, CT 06470-2359
(203) 426-1320

National Skeet Shooting Association/
National Sporting Clays Association
P.O. Box 680007
San Antonio, TX 78268

National Spinal Cord Injury Association
1032 S. LaGrange Rd.
La Grange, IL 60525
(708) 352-6223

National Wheelchair Athletic Association
(NWAA)
3617 Betty Drive, Suite S.
Colorado Springs, CO 80907
(719) 597-8330

North County Independent Living Center
P.O. Box 1245
Superior, WI 54880

NWAA National Governing Body (NGB)
Chairperson-Air Guns
54 Hazard Ave., #319
Enfield, CT 06082
(203) 741-3961

NWAA NGB Chairman-Archery
Road #2
Box 2043
West Sunbury, PA 16061
(412) 735-4359

National Wheelchair Shooting Federation
54 Hazard Ave., #319
Enfield, CT 06082
(203) 741-3961

Oregon School of the Deaf
999 Locust St. N.E.
Salem, OR
(503) 378-3825

Outdoor Buddies, Inc. (Matches able-bodied
"buddies" with hunters with disabilities)
P.O. Box 37283
Denver, CO 80237
(303) 771-8216

Paralyzed Veterans of America
801 Eighteenth St. N.W.
Washington, DC 20006

Physically Challenged Outdoorsman's Association
3006 Louisiana Ave.
Cleveland, Ohio 44109

Products to Assist the Disabled Sportsman
J.L. Pachner, Ltd.
13 Via Dinola
Laguna Niguel, CA 92677
(714) 363-9831

Project Access
P.O. Box 299
Village Station, NY 10014

Project Access
11899 Baily Drive
Lowell, MI 49331

Recreational Outdoor Adventures for Disabled Students American Red Cross, L.A. Chapter
1200 South Vermont Ave.
Los Angeles, CA 99996

Special Olympics International
1350 New York Ave. N.W.
Suite 500
Washington, DC 20005
(202) 628-3630

Self Help for Hard of Hearing People (SHHH)
11303 Hayden Bluff Lane
Hayden, ID 83835-9585
1-800-423-3047

Society for the Advancement of Travel for the Handicapped
347 Fifth Ave., Suite 610
New York, NY 10016

The Travelin' Talk Network
P.O. Box 3534
Clarksville, TN 37043
(615) 552-6670

United States Amputee Athletic Association
P.O. Box 210709
Nashville, TN 37221
(615) 662- 2323

United States Association for Blind Athletes
33 N. Institute Street
Brown Hall, Suite 015
Colorado Springs, CO 80903
(713) 630-0422

United States Cerebral Palsy Athletic Association
34518 Warren Road, Suite #264
Westland, MI 48185
(313) 425-8961

United States Sporting Clays Association
50 Briar Hollow
Suite 490 East
Houston, TX 77027
(713) 622-8043

Wilderness Inquiry
Suite 327
1313 Fifth Street S.E.
Minneapolis, MN 55414

# Appendix VI
## Adaptive Equipment Manufacturers

The Abledata System
National Rehabilitation Information Center
4407 Eighth Street N.E.
Washington, DC 20017
1-800-34-NARIC, (202) 635-5826 TDD

Access to Recreation, Inc. (Distributor of Adapted Recreation Products)
2509 East Thousand Oaks Blvd.
Suite 430
Thousand Oaks, CA 91362
1-800-634-4351, (805) 498-7535

Achievement Products, Inc.
P.O. Box 547
Mineola, NY 11501
(516) 747-8899

IDEA
1393 Meadowcreek Drive #2
Pewaukee, WI 53072
(414) 691-4248

The Alsto Company (Recreation products)
P.O. Box 1267
Galesburg, IL 61401
1-800-447-0048

Applied Technology for Independent Living (Arm braces)
4732 Nevada Avenue N.
Crystal, MN 55428
(612) 537-6377

Autofold, Inc. (Folding rifle support)
208 Coleman St.
P.O. Box 1063
Gardner, MA 01440-1063
(508) 632-0667

Barnett International (Crossbow equipment)
P.O. Box 934
13447 Byrd Drive
Odessa, FL 33556
1-800-237-4507

Beeman Precision Arms (Precision airguns)
3440 AMO Airway Dr.
Santa Rosa, CA 95403

Benjamin Air Rifles Co.
2600 Chicory Rd.
Racine, WI 53403

Childcraft (Recreation products)
22 Kilmer Road
Edison, NJ 08817
1-800-631-5652, (201) 572-6100

Crossman Air Guns, Inc.
980 Turk Hill Rd.
Fairport, NY 14450

Daisy Manufacturing Co., Inc.
Rogers, AR 72756

Educational Teaching Aids (Recreation products)
441 Carpenter Ave.
Wheeling, IL 60090
(708) 520-2500

Flaghouse (Catalogue of physical education and recreational equipment)
18 West 18th Street
New York, NY 10011
(212) 898-9700

Freehanderson Co. (Rifle support, camera harness)
P.O. Box 4543
Helena, MT 59604
(406) 449-2764

Gander Mountain (Adapted recreational products)
P.O. Box 248 Highway West
Wilmot, WI 53192
1-800-558-9410

Guardian Electric Manufacturing Co. (Solenoids for air pressure shooting systems)
1550 West Carroll Ave.
Chicago, IL 60607
(815) 337-0050

Hammatt Senior Products (Adapted recreational products)
P.O. Box 727
Mount Vernon, WA 98273
(206) 428-5850

Harris Communications (Free catalog of listening, signalers devices and books, videos)
Dept. mf-9204
6541 City West Parkway
Eden Prairie, MN 55344-3248
1-800-825-7858, 1-800-825-9187 TDD,
FAX (612) 946-0924

Harry Lawson Co. (Custom rifle stocks)
3328 W. Richey Blvd.
Tucson, AZ 85716

Horton Crossbow Manufacturing Company (Crossbow equipment, electronic crossbow cocking device)
1325 Waterloo Road
Suffield, Ohio 44260

Innovator of Disability Equipment and Adaptations, Inc.
1393 Meadowcreek Drive, Suite 2
Pewaukee, WI 53072
(414) 691-4248

J.L. Pachner, Ltd. (Free catalog, disabled sportsman products)
13 Via Dinola
Laguna Niguel, CA 92677
(714) 363-9831

Jayfro Corporation (Adapted Equipment)
976 Hartford Road
Waterford, CT 06385
(203) 447-4728

Jesana, Ltd. (Adapted recreational equipment)
P.O. Box 17
Irvington, NY 10533
1-800-443-4728

Lakeshore Curriculum Materials
P.O. Box 6261
Carson, CA 90749
1-800-421-5354

Miles Kimball Company
41 West 8th Ave.
Oshkosh, WI 54906
(414) 231-3800

Nationwide Flashing Signal Systems (Visual alerting devices)
8120 Fenton Street
Silver Springs, MD 20910
(301) 589-6671, (301) 589-5153 TDD, FAX (301) 589-6671

Next Generation, Inc.
Trap-House Sporting Clays (Portable trailer mounted sporting clay)
302 Century Ct.
Franklin, TN 37064
David LeAnna
(615) 794-8990

New Era Transportation (Custom vans for persons with disabilities)
810 Moe Dr.
Akron, Ohio 44310
1-800-NET-VANS

The Right Start Catalog (Adapted products)
Right Start Plaza
5334 Sterling Center Drive
Westlake Village, CA 91361
1-800-548-8531

Roleez (All terrain cart)
5711A Sellger Drive
Norfolk, VA 23502
1-800-347-2278 or (804) 461-1122

SR-77 Enterprises
c/o R.W. Bowen
363 Maple Street
Chadron, NE 69337
(308) 432-2894

Things from Bell (Adapted products)
230 Mechanic Street
P.O. Box 206
Princeton, WI 54968
1-800-543-1458

Therapeutic Recreation Systems
1280 28th St. Suite #3
Boulder, CO 80303-1797
(303) 444-4720
(800) 621-8385 ext. 150

T.I.E. Production (Video of concepts and inventions)
P.O. Box 642361
Northwest Station
Omaha, NE 68164

Tru-Fire Corporation (Archery releases)
723 State Street
North Fond du Lac, WI 54935
(414) 923-6866

UNI-USA (Mountain goat cart)
8025 S.W. 185th
Aloha, OR 97007
(503) 649-7922

Wheelers Accessible Van Rentals
Nationwide Rentals
1-800-456-1371

Wilderness Enterprises (Modified sporting equipment)
4634 Embarrass Road
Embarrass, MN 55732
(218) 984-3002

World Magnetics (Pressure/vacuum air switches)
810 Hastings Street
Traversa City, MI 49684
(616) 946-3800

Yankee Medical (Seats for snowmobiles and ATVs)
276 North Ave.
Burlington, VT 05402-1486
Roger Blanchard
1-800-649-4591

# Appendix VII
## Publications

Ability
P.O. Box 37078
Miami, FL 33137

Access America
Suite 501
1111 - 18th Street N.W.
Washington, DC 20036-3894

Beginning Reading and Sign Language Video
T-J Publishers
817 Silver Springs Ave.
Silver Springs, MD 20910

California Parks Access
Cougar Press Publishing
1-800-735-3805
State and National Park Guide
for visitors with limited mobility

Center Shot
NWAA's Airgun Sport Section
269 Stony Hill Rd., T-28
Wilbraham, MA 01095

ChallengeAmerica Chronicle
P.O. Box 690032
San Antonio, TX 78269-0032

Complete Directory for People with Disabilities
Grey House Publishing
Pocket Knife Square
Lakeville, CT 06039

Compuserve-Handicapped Users Database
Computer Bulletin Boards
5000 Arlington Centre Blvd.
Columbus, Ohio 43220
1-800-818-8199

Computer Able Network
P.O. Box 1706
Portland, OR 97207

Design Guide for Accessible Outdoor Recreation
USDA Forest Service
201 - 14th Street S.W.
Washington, DC 20250

Disabled Boaters and Campers News
P.O. Box 173
Lyons, IL 60534

Disabled Outdoors Magazine
2052 West 23rd Street
Chicago, IL 60608
(708) 358-4160

Disability Rights Guide
by Charles Goldman
Media Publishing
2440 O Street Suite 202
Lincoln, NE 69510-1125

Easy Access to National Parks,
the Sierra Club Guide for People with Disabilities
730 Polk Street
San Francisco, CA 94109

Exceptional Parent Magazine
1170 Commonwealth Ave
Boston, MA 02134-9942

Extend Their Reach
Electronic Industries Association
Consumer Electronics Group
2001 Pennsylvania Ave, NW
Washington, DC 20006-1813
(202) 457-4919

Free Spirit News
P.O. Box 560186
Miami, FL 33256
(305) 388-2574

Handbook for the Design of Barrier-Free
Recreational Boating and Fishing Facilities
SOBA
P.O. Box 25655
Washington, DC 20007

Hunter Education Instructor
P.O. Box 19000
Seattle, WA 98109
(206) 624-3845

Mobility Guide
Traffic Safety and Engineering Department
American Automobile Association
1000 AAA Drive
Heathrow, FL 32746-5063

Moving Forward
P.O. Box 3553
Torrance, CA 90510
(310) 320-8793

National Archery Association Publication
Wheelchair Archery Information
1750 East Boulder St.
Colorado Springs, CO 80909-5778
(303) 578-4576

New Mobility Magazine
P.O. Box 4162
Boulder, CO 80306-9906

Outdoors Forever (Newsletter)
P.O. Box 4811
East Lansing, MI 48826
(517) 337-5018

Palaestra: The Forum of Sport,
Physical Education, and
Recreation for the Disabled
P.O. Box 508
Macomb, IL 61455

The Partner
The Bulletin of Capable Partners, Inc.
P.O. Box 47942
Plymouth, MN 55447-0942

Society for the Advancement
of Travel for the Handicapped
347 Fifth Ave., Suite 610
New York, NY 10016

Sports and Recreation for the
Disabled: A Resource Handbook
Benchmark Press, Inc.
8435 Keystone Crossing
Suite 175
Indianapolis, IN 46240

Sports 'N Spokes Magazine
5201 North 19th Ave. Suite 111
Phoenix, AZ 85015
(602) 246-9426

The Travelin' Talk Network and Newsletter
P.O. Box 3534
Clarksville, TN 37043
(615) 552-6670

Uniform Federal Accessibility Standards
General Service Administration
8th and F Street N.W.
Room 3044
Washington, DC 20405
(202) 566-0038

Wyoming Wildlife Magazine
5400 Bishop Blvd
Cheyenne, WY 82006
1-800-548-9453
Now available to people with visual
impairments on special audio cassette.

# Appendix VIII
## Often Used Sign Language and Finger Spelling

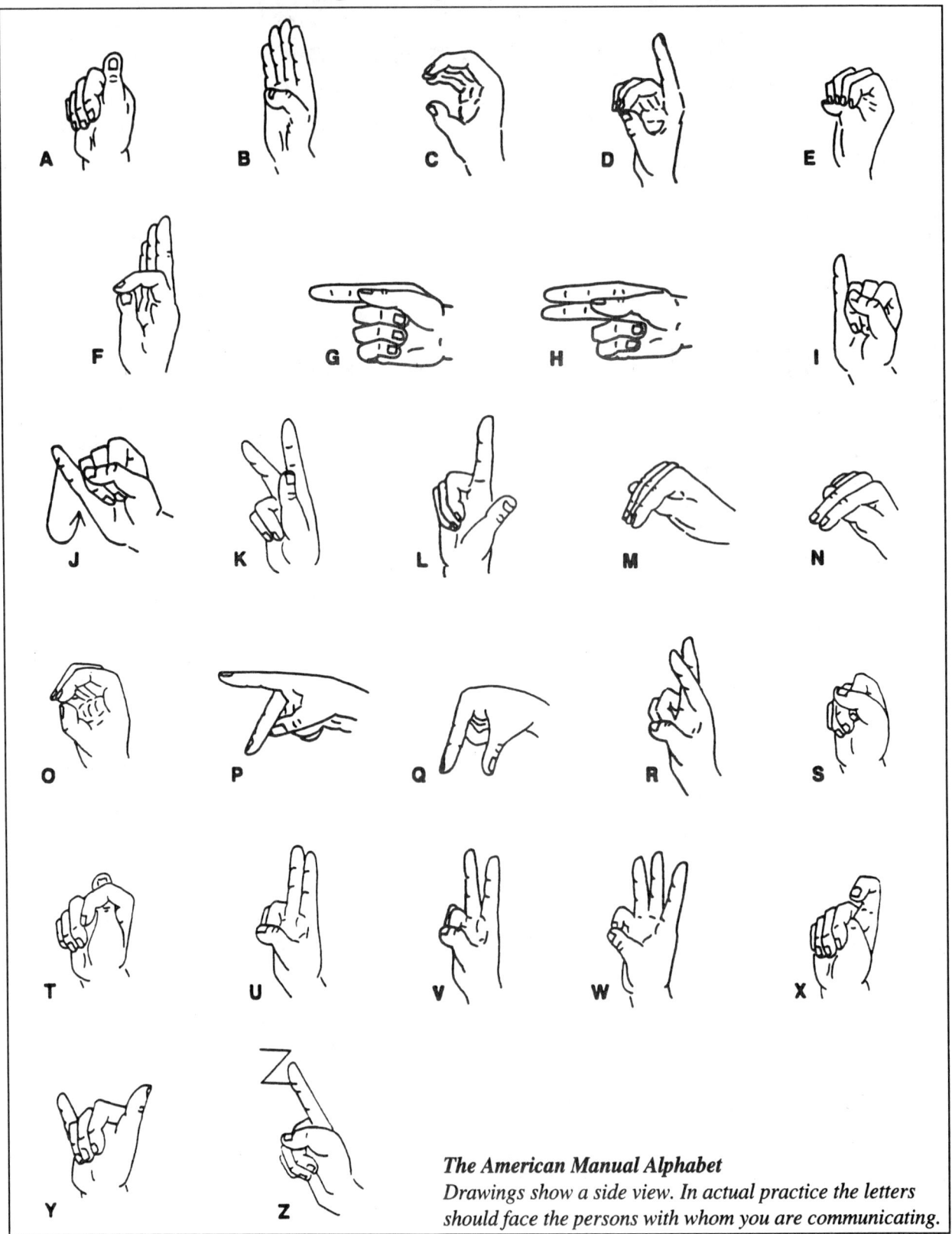

A B C D E
F G H I
J K L M N
O P Q R S
T U V W X
Y Z

*The American Manual Alphabet*
*Drawings show a side view. In actual practice the letters should face the persons with whom you are communicating.*

# Glossary
## Shooting Sports Terms

**A**

**Action:** The part of a firearm that loads, fires and ejects a bullet or shot.
**Ammunition:** Any powder, shot, cartridge or shotshell used in a firearm.
**Automatic:** Firearm which loads, fires and ejects ammunition continuously with one trigger squeeze. Often confused with semi-automatic. Machine guns are true automatics.

**B**

**Ballistics:** Modern science dealing with the motion and impact of projectiles, especially those discharged from firearms.
**Barrel:** The metal tube that the bullet or shot goes down when a firearm is fired.
**Binoculars:** Field glasses used to identify game by making it look larger.
**Black powder:** Granulated powder made of charcoal, sulfur and salt peter; used in muzzleloaders. (See Pyrodex).
**Bolt:** A steel, rod-like assembly which moves back and forth in the action, sealing the cartridge in the chamber during firing.
**Bolt action:** A type of firearm that loads and unloads by working the bolt.
**Bore:** The hollow area inside the barrel that the bullet or shot moves through. The bore's inside measurement determines the caliber or gauge of the firearm.
**Bow:** Device for shooting arrows. Types include straight limb, recurve and compound.
**Bowhunting:** Hunting with bows and arrows.
**Bowstring:** The string on a bow.
**Bow stringer:** Piece of heavy test nylon with a leather pouch at both ends used for stringing a bow.
**Break action:** A type of firearm that opens at the breech. Shells are loaded by hand. This kind can come either as a single-barrel or a double barrel.
**Breech:** The part of a barrel at the end opposite to the muzzle.
**Broadhead:** An arrowhead with two or more razor sharp cutting edges used in hunting.
**Buck shot:** A large size of shot.

**C**

**Caliber:** The measurement of a rifle or handgun bore. Usually, it is the distance between the lands.
**Carrying positions:** Safe ways in which to carry a firearm. Positions include double-hand (ready carry), cradle carry, elbow carry, shoulder carry and sling carry.
**Cartridge:** A container for ammunition which holds primer, powder and the bullet or shot.
**Case:** Container which holds primer, powder and the bullet or shot.
**Centerfire:** Ammunition in which the primer is contained in the center of the base.
**Chamber:** The inside rear part of the barrel where the cartridge is held ready for firing.
**Choke:** The part of a shotgun at the muzzle that controls the spread of the shot and its pattern.
**Clip:** Container which holds ammunition and is attached to the action of a firearm.
**Compass:** Instrument for showing direction, especially one consisting of a magnetic needle swinging freely on a pivot and pointing to the magnetic north.
**Code of ethics:** A set of unwritten rules based on respect for what is safe and fair.
**Conservation:** The wise use of resources.
**Contour lines:** Lines on topographic maps that show the height of hills, slope contours and terrain features.
**Cylinder:** Part of a revolver in which cartridges are loaded or placed.

**D**

**Discharge:** Act of a firearm being fired or going off.
**Dominant eye:** Eye that gives better information to the brain than the other. Also called *master eye*.
**Draw weight:** How many pounds of force it takes to draw the bowstring a certain distance.

**F**

**Firearms:** Tools which shoot projectiles by burning gunpowder.
**Firing pin:** Metal which strikes the primer of ammunition, starting the firing process.
**Flask:** Container used to carry black powder, not to load it.
**Fletching:** Feathers or plastic at the rear of an arrow that help the arrow fly straight.
**Flint:** Rocks that will spark when struck against steel.
**Flintlock:** A gunlock in which a flint in the hammer strikes a metal plate to produce a spark that ignites the powder.
**Forearm:** The front end of the gun stock that is under the barrel.
**Fouling:** A pasty deposit left in the barrel each time a firearm is shot.
**Frame:** The metal housing that gives a handgun its shape.
**Frizzen:** A piece of metal which creates sparks when struck by the flint. This ignites the powder in the flashpan and fires a flintlock muzzleloader.
**Fulminate of mercury:** Explosive used to ignite gunpowder in early firearms. Ignition begins with a sharp blow to the explosive.

**G**

**Gauge:** The size of the bore of a shotgun. It is measured by the number of lead balls the size of the bore which weigh one pound.

**H**

**Half cock:** Certain point between having the firearm hammer in a firing position and in a down position.
**Hammer:** Part of the action which strikes the firing pin, causing the ignition of ammunition.
**Hammer safety:** A type of shotgun safety. It is a small device that stops the firearm from firing if the trigger is pulled accidentally.
**Handgun:** Firearm having a short barrel and which is usually held at arm's length, rather than at the shoulder, to fire.
**Hangfire:** Delay in ignition.
**Hunter orange:** Fluorescent orange color which, when worn by hunters, has helped to decrease the number of hunting accidents.
**Hunter's code:** A set of unwritten rules based on respect for what is safe and fair.

**I**

**Ignition:** Setting fire to the propellant or powder charge.

**L**

**Land:** The metal between the grooves in a rifled barrel.
**Lock:** Firing assembly of a firearm.
**Long starter:** Wood or metal rod used to push the ball and patch down the barrel of a muzzleloader.

## M

**Magazine:** Part of a repeating firearm which holds ammunition until it is ready to be fed into the chamber.
**Magnum:** A type of shotshell or cartridge that has more powder than a standard shotshell.
**Marksmanship:** Skill in placing a shot or hitting a target.
**Master eye:** Eye which gives better information to the brain than the other. Also called *dominant eye*.
**Matchlock:** Oldest style muzzleloader and most elementary form of the rifle.
**Maxi ball:** Lead projectile used in muzzleloaders. Has a solid base which delivers greater weight for a given bore than with a minie ball or round.
**Minie ball:** Lead projectile used in muzzleloaders. Invented to offer easier loading for military use.
**Misfire:** Failure to fire.
**Muzzle:** The end of the barrel where the fired projectile exits.
**Muzzleloader:** A firearm that is loaded through the muzzle instead of the breech.

## N

**Nipple:** Part of percussion cap muzzleloaders which holds the percussion cap. When the cap is struck by the hammer, the ignition process is started.
**Nock:** The slot on an arrow where it fits onto the bowstring.

## P

**Pattern:** Density and scattering of shot pellets when fired. Patterns are affected by choke.
**Pellets:** Small, round balls of lead or steel that are shot in a pattern.
**Percussion:** Oldtime arm which uses a small, metal cap filled with explosives. The cap is placed on the nipple under the hammer and when hit, the cap explodes, sending the flame to the main powder charge which fires the firearm.
**Percussion cap:** Cap placed over a muzzleloader's nipple. When struck with the hammer, fire from the cap ignites the powder in the barrel.
**Peripheral vision:** The ability to see objects out of the corners of the eyes.
**Point:** Sharp end on an arrow. Types include conical, blunt or broadhead.
**Powder:** A rapidly burning material found in centerfire and rimfire ammunition which turns into gas to create enough pressure to fire the bullet or shot.
**Primer:** An explosive cap used to ignite the powder when struck with a sharp blow from the firing pin.
**Priming powder:** The gunpowder used to set off the charge in a gun.
**Projectile:** A bullet or shot that is pushed out of a firearm by force.
**Prone:** Lying flat; the safest and most accurate of the four rifle positions.
**Pump action:** A type of firearm that loads and unloads ammunition by pumping the firearm between shots.
**Pyrodex™:** Chemical substitute for black powder. (See *black powder*.)

## Q

**Quiver:** Container for arrows.

## R

**Ramrod:** Wood or metal rod used to push the ball and patch down the barrel of a muzzleloader.
**Recoil:** The sudden backwards movement of a firearm when fired.
**Repeater:** A firearm that holds more than one cartridge and can fire several shots before reloading.

**Revolver:** A firearm having a revolving cylinder.
**Rifling:** Grooves in the metal of the bore of a firearm which make the bullet spin.
**Rim-fire:** A type of ammunition in which the primer is around the inside bottom rim of the case.

## S

**Safety:** A mechanism designed to stop the firearm from firing accidentally.
**Semi-automatic:** A firearm that fires, ejects the spent cartridge and chambers a new cartridge with a single pull of the trigger.
**Shell:** Container which holds shot and other parts of ammunition for shotguns.
**Short starter:** Short rod used to press the patched ball just into the muzzle when loading a muzzleloader.
**Shot:** Pellets made of lead or steel that are fired by a firearm.
**Shotgun shell:** Also commonly referred to as shotshell, consists of the shot, wad, powder and primer within a case.
**Sight-in:** To adjust a rifle's sights so that the bullet hits a target area at a given range.
**Sights:** Mechanical parts of a firearm which help in aiming. Includes open, peep and telescope.
**Sliding lever:** A type of shotgun safety. It is a small device designed to stop the firearm from firing if the trigger is pulled accidentally.
**Smoothbore:** Firearm without rifling in the bore, usually a shotgun.
**Solvent:** A liquid that can dissolve grease and other substances that can build up inside a firearm.
**Sportsman or sportswoman:** A hunter who obeys all the written and unwritten rules and regulations. A hunter who enjoys the total hunting experience.
**Sprue:** Small, flat side on a muzzleloader ball.
**Stock:** The wooden or plastic frame that holds the barrel and action. It helps you get and keep aim and it absorbs recoil when you fire.

## T

**Trigger:** Mechanical device that starts the firing process on a firearm.
**Trigger guard:** Part of a firearm that protects the trigger from accidentally being released.

## W

**Wheel lock:** Early muzzleloader with a grooved wheel wound tight by a spring to produce sparks. When sparks shoot into the pan, they ignite the powder.
**Wildlife management:** Wise use and manipulation of renewable wildlife resources. It is a field of study based on scientific fact.

## Z

**Zone of fire:** Direction in which each hunter in a group will fire, to be agreed upon before beginning a hunt.

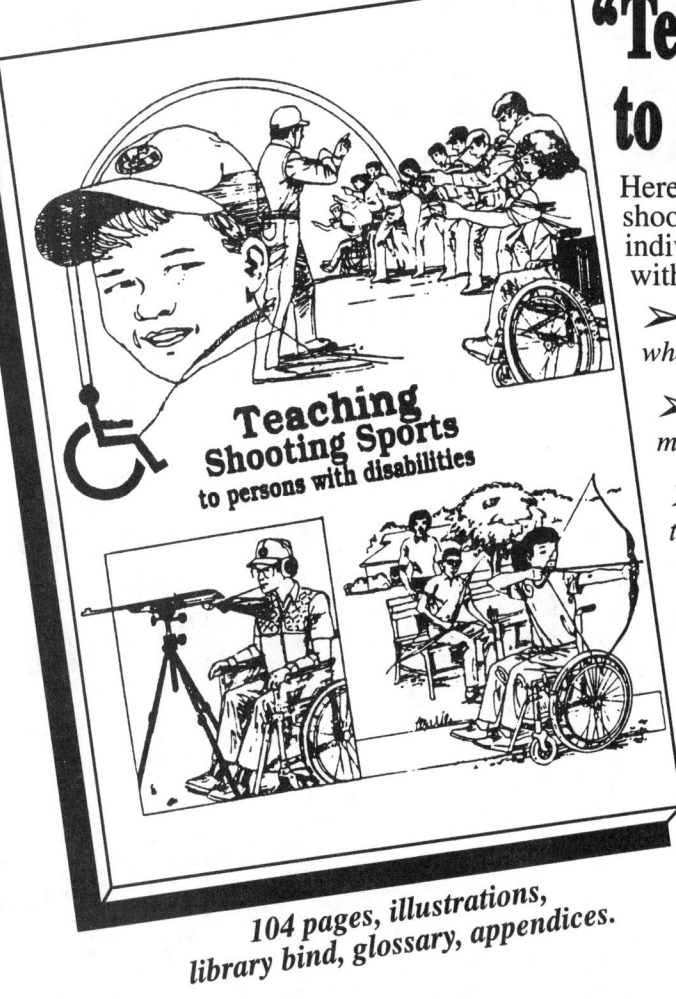

# "Teaching Shooting Sports to persons with disabilities"

Here is the most useful publication available for shooting ranges, clubs, firearms dealers and individual instructors who serve persons with disabilities.

➤ *Be able to recognize various levels of ability, and what limitations each level places on an individual.*

➤ *Gain knowledge on instructing students with physical, mental, learning, hearing and visual impairments.*

➤ *Learn how to be aware of some needs related to specific impairments.*

➤ *Gain skills in assisting people with disabilities overcoming environmental obstacles.*

➤ *Recognize common sense steps to assure safe range conditions for students and instructors.*

➤ *Learn about Rifle/Airgun, Shotgun and Archery assistive devices to help shooters overcome their disabilities for various levels of shooting.*

ISBN: 0-916682-668

*104 pages, illustrations, library bind, glossary, appendices.*

➤ *Build and tailor effective classes and activities for all students using the lesson plans and teaching tips provided.*

➤ *Use the Appendices support information and resources to enhance your classes and activities.*

## Price List

| Quantity | Unit Price | Per Order Shipping Cost |
|---|---|---|
| 1 | $11.95 | Included |
| 2-9 | $9.95 | $3.70 |
| 10-24 | $8.95 | $5.35 |
| 25-49 | $7.95 | $9.35 |
| 50-99 | $6.95 | $17.30 |

Prices effective 1/94. Subject to change without notice.

## ORDER FORM

**Teaching Shooting Sports to persons with disabilities**

Name _____
Title _____
Company _____
Street Address _____
City _____ State _____ Zip _____
Phone ( ___ ) _____ FAX ( ___ ) _____

**Phone Orders call Toll Free 1-800-645-5489
or FAX your order: 206-340-9816**

Mail orders to: Outdoor Empire Publishing, Inc.
511 Eastlake Avenue East • Seattle, WA 98109

| Please Ship | Quantity | Unit Price | Total Price |
|---|---|---|---|
| Books | | $ ea. | $ |
| **Please call for quantities above 99.** | Sub Total | | $ |
| | Add 8.2% Sales Tax WA res. only | | $ |
| | Plus shipping: FOB Seattle, WA | | |
| | **TOTAL** | | $ |

☐ CHECK OR MONEY ORDER ENCLOSED  ☐ VISA  ☐ MasterCard

CREDIT CARD NUMBER
☐☐☐☐ ☐☐☐☐ ☐☐☐☐ ☐☐☐☐

SIGNATURE _____

EXPIRATION DATE  Month __ Year __  P.O. # _____
(Attach original)